HELPING HILDA

Hospital Survival Handbook

Hilda's Daughters
Terry Rudd, RN, MSN
Trish Billings
Linda Cooper

Copyright 2004

This book is dedicated to the memory of our beloved mother, Hilda, who provided the inspiration for our lives and this book. We wish to carry on her lifelong career in healing and hope this book will assist those who are not equipped with the knowledge to cope with illness and hospitalization.

Edited by Caroline Hinckley, M.A. and Ellen Zimet, M.Ed
Cover Photography and design by Brett Langford
Proof Reading and back cover synopsis by Julia Lombardo.

Library of Congress Control Number: 2005900108

ISBN: 0-9759171-0-2

www.helpinghilda.com
1-877-HILDA55
1-877-445-3255

Authors' Notes

We wrote this book to help those people who need to learn how to become advocates and better navigate the medical system. In doing so, we give you the power and permission to observe, ask and intervene on behalf of your family member or friend.

The book took us about two years to write and was begun when our mother was still alive. We didn't know that her hospitalization would be the beginning of her final journey and had hoped to have her as an active participant in our writing. We were helped along the way by persons who were interested in "getting the word out" about advocating for those who were hospitalized. Many times during this process, rough drafts of the book were sent to individuals who were assuming a role as advocate and needed the information right away.

The enthusiastic responses from individuals confirmed that this book was necessary and timely. All who utilized the information, even those in the medical field, stated the book was necessary and had helped them in some way to work through a hospital or care facility crisis.

We would sincerely like to thank our editors, Caroline Hinckley, M.A., and Ellen Zimet, M.Ed., who worked selflessly, met with us on numerous occasions, and re-wrote much of the information in a friendly format for a non-medical audience. Caroline was especially helpful in rewriting the poems to give them proper meter and flow. Interestingly enough, in the course of the re-writing, Ellen found the need to use the information from this book to advocate for a family member who needed emergency treatment and surgery.

Thanks and appreciation is also given to Julia Lombardo who helped with the synopsis of the book. A special thank you goes to Dr. Ivan Reeve and Liz Reeve. They provided us with valuable medical insights, as well as personal perspectives on how they handled the illness of their son, who became paralyzed from metastatic cancer.

Much thanks goes to the experts who read the book and

gave us their valuable feedback: Jill McGraw, RN, B.V.E., George Cardoso, Flex Ed, Lana Van Sant RN; Mary Anne McGinley, M.Ed.; Ivan Reeve, M.D.; Liz Reeve, Author; David Steinberger, PhD., Psychologist and Andrea Hamilton, CPT. We would also like to thank those persons who gave us anecdotes and insights into their own experiences, that helped focus the direction of the book. We chose, for this book, to leave the anecdotes as Hilda's, but will include these shared stories in future writings.

Our mother could not have had the quality of life at the end of her life without the love and caring of her caregivers. We sincerely give thanks to Christina Garcia, Jennifer Kaylor, Krissy Hodges, Li Hoang, Susie Bradshaw, Moss, and the wonderful resources of Julie Siri at Comfort Keepers. We are grateful for your service to Hilda that enabled her to be at home during her last days.

We wish that no one will ever have to use this book, but we recommend it be part of your personal library, just in case. We also hope, as a result of reading this book, you will appreciate the remarkable life of our mother, Hilda, and the legacy that will continue as a result of this book.

We intend to add further to Helping Hilda through additional works and a Website. We encourage your suggestions and comments as we develop a repertoire of ideas focused on helping others. Welcome to our Team!

With Love,

Terry, Trish, and Linda

Table of Contents

Prologue

Hilda's Story

Hilda Shaylor, my mother, was not a "stereotypical" 82-year-old woman. She was a vibrant, independent female who lived alone in Laguna Beach, California, one block from the Pacific Ocean. Any time the ocean temperature was over 67 degrees, she went to her local beach, Diver's Cove, to body surf. She was well-tanned and in fit condition.

Having been a registered nurse for over 50 years, Hilda indicated there was never a day she had not loved her work, and in fact, regretted the fact that she retired too soon. But, in retirement, Hilda kept incredibly busy. She owned and managed her own home and finances, volunteered as a docent at the local museum, and drove throughout Southern California to visit family and friends. Many of her friends were decades younger than she and yet had difficulty at times keeping up with her energy level, ideas, sense of humor and plans to live life to the fullest. She had three children, seven grandchildren, and two great grandchildren whom she visited and communicated with on a regular basis.

Hilda, like a cat with nine lives, had survived ovarian cancer, a five-vessel bypass surgery, and spinal cord surgery with minimal side effects. Her recoveries from all these illnesses were speedy and exceeded all expectations. So it appeared to be just another life challenge when my mother called me in early April of 2002 to indicate she had fallen and had been experiencing loss of sensation in her feet. She underwent an MRI that indicated there was a tumor on her spinal cord, and I attended the meeting with Hilda and the neurosurgeon, who indicated that surgery was needed. The neurosurgeon stated there was a five percent chance of paralysis with surgery and probable paralysis without surgery. As she had undergone a similar procedure twenty years earlier, her choice was to proceed with the operation in a desire to resume her lifestyle after recovery.

The day before her surgery, Hilda went body surfing in the ocean with her dear friend, Doris Shields, acting as her lifeguard for this ocean adventure. After her swim, she went home to prepare for her upcoming hospitalization.

On June 17, 2002, Hilda had surgery for removal of a benign tumor from her spinal column. When my sisters, Linda and Trish, and I (Terry) were invited in to the recovery room, we saw her open her eyes, move her legs and then kick them as if she were paddling out to sea. All three of us broke out in wide grins and were thrilled to see that she had made it through the surgery and was definitely not paralyzed. Hilda was in high spirits!

A continual flow of family and friends kept a vigil, checking on Hilda regularly in the neurosurgery intensive care unit (Neuro ICU). The advantage of this intensive care unit is that the nursing staff is assigned no more than two patients, resulting in close monitoring and observation. My sisters and I left multiple home, business and cell phone numbers for staff to reach us if there were any decisions or problems that needed our attention. We wanted staff to know that we were available to them 24 hours a day. The comfort of the ICU care provided us all with a sense that we could resume our schedules as we awaited Hilda's return to full capacity.

However, on June 19, around 10:30 p.m., I received a call from my sister, Linda, indicating that she had heard a message on her answering machine. A nurse had called, stating that Hilda was upset and wanted to see her family. Arriving home, I found a similar message on my machine. When I called the hospital, I was stunned to hear that Hilda had lost sensation in her legs.

I immediately left for the hospital. As a Registered Nurse with background in critical care as well as a nurse educator, I am very knowledgeable about hospital procedures and what the expectations are for each level of care. To my disbelief, I arrived at Hilda's bedside to hear a nurse relate, with seemingly little concern, that my mother had lost sensation below the waist. The nurse seemed coldly complacent and somewhat disinterested in the situation. I could not believe it, because in my mind, this was a neurological emergency! I asked the nurse if Hilda had been seen by her physician, and was told that she had only been seen by the resident on call. I insisted on speaking to a physician.

Only after talking with the resident/intern on call, did Hilda receive additional doses of anti-inflammatory medicine and have a CAT scan ordered. Even though Hilda was in Neuro ICU, no vital signs had been taken for four hours; neither the nurses nor the intern/resident had contacted her physician and no vital medications had been administered that could offset this inflammation. By the time the hospital staff responded, it was 6 hours after the initial onset of paralysis and too late to reverse the effects.

Hilda was kept in Neuro ICU for another three days, where she received observation, IVs and basic supportive care. She was then transferred to the hospital floor, where her basic supportive care was continued.

At the end of eleven days after the surgery, the medical team determined that Hilda's acute hospital stay was concluded, and required us to transfer her to a facility where she would receive spinal cord rehabilitation. The family decided on a well-recognized center that was close to my home, where I could have immediate access to assisting with Hilda's needs.

Unknown to us at that time, the hospital had failed to prepare Hilda medically for transfer to a rehabilitation center. An open bedsore on her buttocks was failing to heal. Her white blood cell count was a dramatically high 19, probably indicating a major infection. As a result, her first two weeks in spinal cord rehab were spent trying to help her stabilize medically.

The family kept trying to make her "get up and go." We all tried to encourage her and push her with activities, but she had no energy and no ability to do anything. Because this facility had an excellent medical staff, they kept close watch on her and informed me that she was nutritionally deprived. I began bringing in protein bars and feeding her as much as I could. Hilda was exhausted and anxious. She began to become emotionally overwrought. She was so frustrated that she couldn't just "walk" and do what she needed to do. This once very active woman resented that she was now fully dependent and became angry and scared that her needs would not be met.

Because her anxiety level was so high, and she began to obsess about suicide, we arranged for full-time care. Although she had two health care policies, long-term care, and supplemental insurance, none of them paid for this extra support. When she realized that we were paying for this care, she became even more distraught.

My sisters and I were doing whatever we could to try to make her life livable. We encouraged her in the rehab center and arranged for additional caregivers, consisting of family, friends and hired agency personnel. These people were the best, encouraging Hilda to joke and display that "cute" aspect of her personality that everyone found so enchanting. Family came from South Africa, England, Hong Kong and other countries to visit with Hilda. To see her in this condition was shocking and painful for everyone. Because she had weathered other operations and illnesses so successfully, everyone continued to believe that Hilda would complete her rehab and soon be doing wheelies in downtown Laguna.

As Hilda continued to weaken, we continued to encourage her. Her white blood count was still high, the bedsore was not healing, and we began to see a brown fluid oozing from her back. Perhaps because she was paralyzed and felt no pain, the seriousness of these symptoms was minimized. The medical team finally ordered blood and skin cultures in an attempt to identify the source of the infection. Once they found she had antibiotic-resistant bacteria in her urine and her wound, an infectious disease doctor was called in for consultation.

Hilda now was placed in isolation, requiring staff to use masks, gloves, and maintain a highly sterile environment. Additionally, the infectious disease doctor called in a wound care specialist to examine Hilda because, although her back wound was sutured, brown ooze continually appeared. The wound care specialist opened her suture and pulled out a dressing that had never been removed. A week later, since the oozing was still occurring, the wound care specialist went back into the area and found a second retained dressing from deep inside her back. At this point, we recognized this may have been the cause of the skin breakdown, high white cell count, invasive bacteria and her exhaustion.

None of us would have suspected that the possible cause of all the agony and paralysis was a retained dressing. The physicians at the spinal cord center immediately tried to contact the neurosurgeons from the original admitting hospital. After three days, the rehab hospital case manager was finally able to contact the neurosurgeon who had performed the operation.

The neurosurgeon asked that she be transferred back to the original facility to be evaluated. Hilda was admitted and continued to deteriorate. The bacteria in her body forced the hospital to keep her in isolation. Her wound continued to deteriorate, and she developed lung problems. Our loving mother was demoralized, depleted and debilitated.

As Hilda's condition at the hospital continued to worsen, she repeatedly indicated she did not want to be resuscitated if her heart were to stop or if she were to stop breathing. In keeping with her wishes, a "no code" was to be attached to her chart. As her designated health care voice, I assumed this request would be honored. I was therefore shocked to accidentally discover that she had been designated a "partial code," indicating that she would be placed on a ventilator if she stopped breathing. Even with the documentation and Hilda's insistence regarding her wishes, the physicians refused to reverse the order. Through my vehement insistence, I was finally successful in restoring a "no code" notation to Hilda's medical chart.

Hilda became severely depressed and wished to go home to her apartment. The hospital environment was very toxic to her, and the treatments were worsening her condition daily. A physician who had experience with hospice care agreed to discharge her, although we were told she would most likely not make it through the next few days, since she suffered from fever, respiratory problems and infection that were ravaging her body.

Even though the directive allowing Hilda to go home was

issued on a holiday, Labor Day, 2002, we made arrangements to move her that very day into her second floor apartment. Hospice was wonderful. In a heartbeat they arranged for a hospital bed, a lift, to help her out of bed, oxygen, if needed, and a wheelchair. I arranged my schedule to stay with Hilda to provide nursing care.

Hilda suffered an additional two days of fever and then started to improve. Over the next few months, we worked slowly on Hilda's recovery. We worked on her nutrition, skin care, flexibility, encouraged her friends to visit and arranged for 24-hour care. We provided adventures by hiring day workers to carry her down the stairs so we could take her to see her beloved ocean and visit the Laguna downtown area. We took her to movies and plays. Hilda was such a sport, enduring the stares of strangers and the accidental bumps that occurred getting her up and down the stairs. The day workers began to know "ilda" by name and offered to help whenever they could.

Throughout this ordeal, my sisters and I each contributed our unique talents. I was the nurse. Linda lived in town and handled all day-to-day chores, and Trish took care of the paperwork and bills. Between the three of us, we were meeting her needs in our own way.

We continued to plan long-term arrangements for Hilda. A former student of mine, who was also a surfer, participated in her care. She moved in next door and we placed a door between the two apartments.

But Hilda became weaker and indicated she did not want to continue to live this way. She said she just couldn't fight anymore. She asked each of us separately if that was all right with us. We all gave her the same answer: "Mom, we will help you live a life to the fullest, but if you really don't want to live this way, we support your decision".

This discussion coincided with Hilda finding out she was severely anemic. We planned to get her some blood transfusions, but she opted to refuse. Over the next week, Hilda deteriorated and then died. Her last breaths were spent with the youngest of her caregivers, Christina. We were able to be with her for the hours after her death, a wonderful time to reminisce and see her progress to a peaceful and smiling face, even in death.

I should say at this time that this situation, for our family, was the worst of times, but also the best of times. We were able to connect with our mother, and my sisters and I found not only how much we all deeply loved our mother but also totally agreed on what we wanted for her. This also gave us time to tell our mother how much we loved her. There were many times that we all held hands around her bed and professed our love for her and each other. Taking her home had given us another six months to be together.

Since Hilda's death, my sisters and I have spent sleepless nights reviewing what we could or should have done differently. How could I have not noticed that my mother had become so nutritionally deficient? Why did I not notice that Hilda was in no condition to be transferred to the rehab hospital? Could we have been more vigilant and omnipresent during her hospital stay?

We also wrestle with additional questions. Why were hospital personnel so ineffectual when Hilda's paralysis occurred while recovering in the Neurological Intensive Care Unit? Why weren't drugs given immediately? Why were we not notified immediately? When, where and by whom were the dressings left in her wound? Why did the hospital staff not recognize her malnutrition? Why was she sent to the rehab hospital when she was still very ill? Why was her white blood cell count ignored or overlooked?

There are even more questions we could ask about our current medical system, its personnel, and the reasons it functions the way it does. I trusted the medical system, and I was wrong. I realized too late that I needed to be with my mother constantly, advocate for her and literally be *joined at the hip* in order to ensure that, in this fractured system, necessary care was provided.

Since we first began thinking, talking and writing about the conditions surrounding our mother's surgery, we have talked to hundreds of people with similar stories who wished they had more information to assist their loved one through a hospitalization ordeal. The purpose of this book is to give you the tools to become an advocate for your loved one as soon as he or she becomes hospitalized. This book seeks to provide you with an understanding of the resources and personnel within the hospital, explanations of terms and medical tests and sets of tasks and procedures you can do for your loved one to aid and comfort him or her.

Our hope is that you develop the base of knowledge to ask the right questions and have the ability to assertively participate in the care of your loved one. If we can prevent Hilda's Story from happening to others, our goal will have been met, and Hilda will have made her final contribution to a world that is better for her having been a part of it.

With Love and Caring,

Hilda's Daughters
Linda Cooper
Trish Billings
Terry Rudd

The Need for Advocacy and Empowerment

In other states and days of old,
Our sick and ill had hands to hold.
We brought them food, and love- our best,
While doctors gave them cures and tests.

But now we've given total care
To those who often are not there.
We stay at home and wonder why
Our loved ones have begun to die.

Our role must be to fight for facts;
To ask and question every act.
To help the sick survive their stay
And live to love another day.

CHAPTER 1
The Need for Advocacy and Empowerment

The American medical system is unique in its approach to treating patients. In other countries, people still rely heavily upon one general practitioner for diagnosis and treatment. In the United States, care is given over to numerous specialists, each responsible for a particular body part or function. Having multiple physicians can result in uncoordinated care and overmedication, because consultation among several physicians every time one of them sees a patient is difficult. As a result, a patient's therapeutic regimen may be changed without the input of the patient's other physicians.

In many other countries, once the individual enters the hospital, the family moves in also. Surrounding the patient with love and support, members of the family provide all the food and basic care, while the role of the medical team is to provide treatment and medications. In the United States, when someone is hospitalized, the entire care is relegated to the medical team. The patient is usually isolated, and family contacts are regulated, minimized, and often limited. Since the medical team in the United States is also geared to the priorities of treatment and medications, basic care is sometimes not the highest priority.

That basic care is often missing is not a rare situation. A leading consumer magazine documented a study and presented the following findings after surveying 21,000 respondents:

- The most important factors in a hospital are sufficient staff, systems for organized care and experience with the medical condition being treated.

- People hospitalized for non-surgical treatment are more at risk for poor care.

- The risk of death is directly related to the nurse's workload.
- Only 60% of respondents felt the hospital was adequately staffed.
- 13% of nursing positions in hospitals are unfilled.
- 3% to 4% of hospitalized patients experience some kind of adverse event.
- 19% of the time, medication errors were made.
- 6% of respondents developed an infection during the hospital stay.
- Up to 49% of respondents indicated inadequate pain relief.

The general thrust of the study indicates a gap between care hospitalized patients should receive versus what they are receiving. It is obvious that family members and friends can step into that gap and serve both as watchdogs to the quality of care the patient receives as well as provide some elements of basic care themselves.

The study suggested the following:

- If more than one hospital is an option, try to research which hospital would be the best.
- Be certain that someone accompanies the patient when they are admitted, to ask and answer questions.
- Provide the patient's medical history so that the hospital staff can be aware of allergies, medications the patient is presently taking, names and addresses of physicians, insurance information, and other important data. (A sample health history form is included in the Appendix.)
- Bring outside help in whenever possible. Hospital staffing is so strained that patients do not get the care that they need. Two percent of respondents hired a private duty nurse or sitter to be there when they could not be there.
- Family members should make an effort to get to know the staff and allow the staff to get to know them.
- Write down all questions for the doctor regarding treatment,

medications, and changes in condition.

- If the patient is unable to ask about medications, try to double-check all medications before they are administered.
- Be assertive about asking for pain relief.
- Help nurses work efficiently by being aware of shift changes, and save questions until the nurse has an opportunity to be updated.
- Keep the frequency of visitors and calls under control. Limit them if necessary.
- Plan the patient's discharge. Make sure you receive a formal discharge plan from the hospital.

Other recommendations for how family members can become actively involved in caring for someone who is hospitalized are contained in subsequent chapters.

It should be remembered that patients have rights. All medical facilities have adopted a Patient Bill of Rights that should be posted and available to all. While that list might vary from facility to facility and state to state, basic rights such as privacy, choice, equal access, decision-making, confidentiality, and non-discrimination should be included.

The following is an example of a patient's Bill of Rights. As with any set of rights, its effectiveness is ensured when individuals are active and vigilant in their enforcement. The strong and healthy can do it for them. The ill and weak will need help.

Sample Patient Bill of Rights

I. Information Disclosure

You have the right to receive accurate and easily understood information about your health plan, health care professionals, and health care facilities. If you speak another language, have a physical or mental disability, or just don't understand something, assistance will be provided so you can make informed health care decisions.

II. Choice of Providers and Plans

You have the right to a choice of health care providers that is sufficient to provide you with access to appropriate high-quality health care.

III. Access to Emergency Services

If you have severe pain, an injury, or sudden illness that convinces you that your health is in serious jeopardy, you have the right to receive screening and stabilization, emergency services whenever and wherever needed, without prior authorization or financial penalty.

IV. Participation in Treatment Decisions

You have the right to know all your treatment options and to participate in decisions about your care. Parents, guardians, family members, or other individuals that you designate can represent you if you cannot make your own decisions.

V. Respect and Nondiscrimination

You have a right to considerate, respectful and nondiscriminatory care from your doctors, health plan representatives, and other health care providers.

VI. Confidentiality of Health Information

You have the right to talk in confidence with health care providers and to have your health care information protected. You also have the right to review and copy your own medical record and request that your physician amend your record if it is not accurate, relevant, or complete.

VII. Complaints and Appeals

You have the right to a fair, fast, and objective review of any complaint you have against your health plan, doctors, hospitals or other health care personnel. This includes complaints about waiting times, operating hours, the conduct of health care personnel, and the adequacy of health care facilities.

The Patient's Bill of Rights includes many choices for the

patient. Look at these carefully. When you have a strong feeling that something is going wrong, a timely consultation or transfer of facilities may save a life. A complaint and appeal may be too little, too late.

Speak Up: Help Prevent Errors in Your Care

Hospitals are on a mission to help patients speak up more about their care. In March 2002, The Joint Commission on Accreditation of Healthcare Organizations (JCAHO), together with the Centers for Medicare and Medicaid Services (CMS), launched a national program to urge patients to take a role in preventing health care errors by becoming active, involved and informed participants on the health care team. The program features brochures, posters and buttons with the *Speak Up*[SM] message:

- **S**peak up if you have questions or concerns, and if you don't understand, ask again. It's your body and you have a right to know.

- **P**ay attention to the care you are receiving. Make sure you're getting the right treatments and medications by the right health care professionals. Don't assume anything.

- **E**ducate yourself about your diagnosis, the medical tests you are undergoing, and your treatment plan.

- **A**sk a trusted family member or friend to be your advocate.

- **K**now what medications you take and why you take them. Medication errors are the most common health care errors.

- **U**se a hospital, clinic, surgery center, or other type of health care organization that has undergone a rigorous on-site evaluation against established state-of-the-art quality and safety standards, such as that provided by JCAHO.

- **P**articipate in all decisions about your treatment. You are the center of the health care team.

The American Nurses Association also supports *Speak*

Up. "Such questioning is particularly important with regard to inadequate staffing and nursing shortages…With the dangers that short staffing poses to patients, no patient should enter a medical facility without knowing whether there will be enough qualified staff on hand to provide adequate care. Every patient has a right to know whether he or she will be assigned an RN, how many RNs are on duty and whether any RNs are working overtime."

The American Nurses Association suggests additional questions patients should be asking about the quality of their nursing care:

- Will I be assessed and monitored throughout my stay or procedure by an RN?

- How many patients are assigned to each RN on my care unit, during the day, at night and on weekends?

- What other health care personnel will be working with my RN? What are their qualifications and what tasks will they perform?

- Does the facility rely on temporary nurses during staffing shortages?

- Does the facility require nurses to work mandatory overtime, and, if so, for how long beyond the regularly scheduled shift?

- Is my nurse regularly assigned and fully oriented to this unit/specialty area?

- Will an RN brief me on follow-up care?

If patients are not satisfied with the responses they get to their inquiries – or if they believe they have received poor care or unsafe staffing – they should contact their state health agency or JCAHO.

We too often believe that speaking up will alienate the staff from the patient and threaten the quality of care. As a nurse, I have not seen staff respond adversely when patients speak up about their care. The patient's medical team needs to know what questions you have, what misconceptions you may have, and how the team can be of assistance. Speaking up is a <u>skill</u>

to be practiced when advocating for the patient.

JCAHO also helps track actions that are called Sentinel Events because they signal the need for immediate investigation and response. A sentinel event is an unexpected occurrence involving death or serious physical or psychological injury. Serious injury specifically includes loss of limb or function.

A summary of the 2003 Sentinel Events can help you see which settings may be at highest risk for events, and which events are most prevalent. If the patient is involved in a procedure that may involve one of these potential events, you may be able to prevent a problem by providing additional vigilance and advocacy.

JCAHO reviewed 2,405 sentinel events since January 1995. The total number of events reported has increased from 23 in 1995 to 487 in 2003. Of the sentinel events reported, 75% resulted in death and 10% in loss of function. Sources for sentinel events could be self-reporting, the media, patient complaints, items identified during surveys and reports provided from state agencies. The number and type of sentinel event, its percentage of the total and the location where it occurred are summarized in the following charts.

General Hospital

Event	#	%
Op/Post-op Complication	296	19.0
Wrong-Site Surgery	274	17.6
Medication Error	229	14.7
Suicide	84	5.4
Delay in Treatment	78	5.0

Hospital – Emergency Department

Event	#	%
Delay in Treatment	50	51.5
Medication Error	12	12.4
Suicide	9	9.3
Restraint-related Event	4	4.1
Assault/rape/homicide	3	3.1

Psychiatric Hospitals

Event	#	%
Suicide	143	46.6
Restraint-related event	39	12.7
Assault/rape/homicide	26	8.5
Elopement (leaving the hospital against advice)	14	4.6
Medication Error	11	3.6

Long-Term Care Facilities

Event	#	%
Patient Fall	21	25.3
Ventilator Death	9	10.8
Assault/Rape/Homicide	8	9.6
Elopement (leaving the hospital against advice)	8	9.6
Suicide	7	8.4

Home Care

Event	#	%
Fire	21	42.9
Medication Error	7	14.3
Patient Fall	3	6.1
Ventilator Death	3	6.1
Medical Equipment Related	2	4.1

Since the overwhelming majority of sentinel events occurs in hospitals, selecting quality health care services for you, a relative or friend requires special thought and attention. JCAHO has prepared information to assist you in knowing what to look for and what to ask.

Your choice of medical providers and hospitals is based upon the nature of the illness and where the physician may practice. If you are drawn to a specific physician or hospital, your choices for the best care possible may be limited. Other times, your choice of medical facility is taken out of your hands when an emergency or unexpected event lands you in a facility that is out of your community or state.

As an advocate for the patient, it is important to know that you can request a different facility or physician if the situation warrants a change. An appropriate mix of physician, hospital, and medical care is essential to getting the best care possible.

Begin by asking your physician about the advantages or special characteristics of each hospital where he or she practices. Your physician can help you select the hospital that is best for you. You should also verify which hospitals are accepted by your insurance, HMO or PPO plan. Then ask the following questions to help you determine which hospital meets your needs.

General Information

Is the hospital accredited by a nationally recognized accrediting body, such as the Joint Commission? Joint Commission accreditation means the organization voluntarily sought accreditation and met national health and safety standards. The Joint Commission provides on-site surveys to review the hospital's medical and nursing care, physical condition, life safety program, special care units, pharmaceutical services, infection control procedures and a number of other areas affecting patient care.

Is the hospital clean? Visit the hospital and look around. Ask to see the waiting rooms and patient care rooms. Does the waiting room look comfortable? Would you want to recuperate in the patient rooms? Do the patient rooms have comfortable chairs for visitors? Do you have privacy in the room?

Your Specific Needs

Do the services and specialties provided by the hospital meet your specific medical needs? Do you have a medical condition requiring specialized attention? Your medical history and present medical condition may affect the type of hospital you choose.

Does the hospital explain the patient's rights and responsibilities? Ask to see a copy of the hospital's patient rights and responsibilities information.

Do you know who is responsible for maintaining your personal care plan? How are the involved practitioners kept informed about your specific care needs? Can you or your family be kept up-to-date on your medical care?

Does the hospital have social workers? Ask what services the social workers provide. Social workers usually help patients and their families find emotional, social, clinical, physical and financial support services.

Discharge Planning

Will a discharge plan be developed for you before you leave the hospital? Ask what services are available and what your primary care physician's involvement will be.

Does the hospital provide you with the necessary training to continue your care in your home after you have been discharged? Ask what training is provided in changing dressings, taking medications or using medical devices. Does the hospital provide you with easy-to-understand written instructions?

Bedside Story

Hilda was a self-sufficient person who was well able to speak for herself. As a family, we felt a need to be close to her after her surgery, and we stayed with her during the 24 hours after surgery. As Hilda seemed to be doing well, we went to our respective homes with the intent of seeing her the next day. We should have continued to be close to her side. Hilda became paralyzed and the nurse on duty only left messages that our mother "was anxious". The nurse also failed to get Hilda immediate medical attention for her paralysis.

The nursing staff failed in their diligence to contact the family and the medical team when Hilda's condition deteriorated. When I look back at the errors that are likely to occur in hospitals, Hilda experienced two sentinel events-post-operative complications and delay in treatment.

After these events occurred and complications arose, we quickly reassessed mechanisms through which the hospital staff could reach us, and developed rotating shifts in order to stay close to our mother. Even so, we miscalculated the continued lack of care that was given to Hilda. The medical team, in their rush to have Hilda transferred to rehabilitation, overlooked her continued medical deterioration. As a result, Hilda was discharged prematurely.

To help prevent these occurrences, family and friends can develop mechanisms to make it very clear to the medical team how the family can be reached. It is best to identify one person as the lead contact who will then disseminate information to other family members. When your loved one is ill, remember that his or her regular defenses are diminished. Even if that person has been the strongest member in the family and has always been a good decision-maker, when hospitalized, an advocate needs to be close by to monitor care and decisions.

*Key Points

- Identify one person as the primary contact.
- Give yourself permission to be actively involved in the care.
- Speak Up when there are concerns.
- Educate yourself about the areas where errors are most likely to occur.
- Do a quick survey of the hospital so you have an idea of the challenges ahead and so you may anticipate areas of concern.

Notes

_____

_____

_____

_____

_____

_____

_____

_____

_____

_____

_____

_____

_____

_____

_____

_____

_____

_____

Communicating Information

I know some things as next of kin
About the person checking in.
The allergies and meds he takes,
The trips to far out lands he makes.

The records of his recent ills
Old surgeries, and spells, and spills.
This info you should take as news
And serve as diagnostic clues.

The doctors need to know as well
Just whom to notify and tell.
The legal role that you do play,
And if you have the final say.

CHAPTER 2
Communicating Information

There is a school of thought in medicine that the best diagnoses can be made by getting a good health history and talking with the patient. The physical examination and diagnostic testing supports that which was obtained in the patient history. The more information the medical team has at its fingertips, the better treatment your loved one can receive. Medical history and ongoing history and communication can be more important than many other tools of medicine combined. It is helpful to have this information ahead of time, in writing, and in the hands of your loved one and yourself.

This chapter contains samples of the types of information that you need to provide the medical team and/or have in your possession in order to make decisions for the patient if he or she cannot. You should think of preparing these forms as "hospital readiness."

The first essential document is a medical history. This form includes the following:

(1) The patient's personal information;
(2) Emergency contact information and the names and phone numbers of relatives;
(3) Medical history, including previous illnesses, hospitalizations and surgeries;
(4) Food and drug allergies;
(5) Current medications;
(6) Normal level of activity;
(7) Current medical concerns, including possible exposures to disease.

Health care providers can give much better care if they have access to a patient's medical history. For example, the medications a patient takes may serve as clues to the nature of the medical problem; it should be noted that many medications are used to treat more than one ailment. A current medical history that contains a list of what medications the patient is currently taking removes the need for guesswork and can certainly contribute to accurate diagnosis and treatment. When in the hospital, keep the history close to the bedside so different members of the medical team can access it. It is also suggested that patients try to get all their medications from the same pharmacy. An alert pharmacist can look for duplications or for drugs that will interact negatively with one another.

Below is a sample of a medical history form. A blank one can be found in Appendix A.

PERSONAL DATA

Name   Hilda Shaylor
Address   555 Main Street, Anyplace,
                              USA 55555
Telephone   (555) 123-4567
Work Phone   Cell Phone (555) 456-1234

Occupation   Retired Nurse. Works as a
Docent
Health Plan Name: Medicare
Health Plan Number: 555-55-5555
Health Plan Phone: (800) 555-6789
Emergency Contact Name: Terry Rudd (Daughter)
Emergency Contact Phone: Call Cell First (555) 122-2345

If no live response, call home (555) 456-7890

If no live response, call my work (555) 555-6789

In an emergency, DO NOT JUST LEAVE A MESSAGE. Call alternate numbers.

Name and Phone Number of Key Individuals (Family, friends, significant others)

Person's Name	Relationship	Telephone
Linda Cooper	Daughter	555-555-5555
Trish Billings	Daughter	555-555-5555
Doris Smith	Friend	555-555-5555
Katy Jones	Friend	555-555-5555
Marion Myers	Friend	555-555-5555

Physician(s) Name and Phone Number

Physician Name	Specialty	Telephone
Dr. John Smith	Cardiology	555-555-5555
Dr. Mary Jones	Internist	555-555-5555
Dr. D. Shah	Oncologist	555-555-5555
Dr. Mary Myers	Gynecologist	555-555-5555

Medical History: Previous Illnesses, Hospitalizations, and Surgeries

Family History (blood relatives)
Mother   Deceased age 78, Diabetes
Father   Deceased age 92, Asthma, fractured hip
Brother(s) 72, alive, no major health problems
Sister(s) age 13 deceased - Epilepsy

Previous Illnesses and Operations	Year Diagnosed	Status Resolved or Continues
Ovarian Cancer	1988	Resolved
Coronary Artery Bypass – 5 grafts	1992	Resolved
Atrial Fibrillation	1992	Continues

Hospitalization Reason	Date	Place	Length of Stay
Spinal Meningioma	1980	Main Street Hospital	2 weeks
Ovarian Tumor Removed	1998	Grand Ave Hospital	12 days
Coronary Artery Bypass	1992	Grand Ave Hospital	2 weeks

Surgery Reason	Date	Place
Spinal Meningioma	1980	Main Street Hospital
Ovarian Tumor Removed	1998	Grand Ave Hospital
Coronary Artery Bypass	1992	Grand Ave Hospital

Recent Travel: 2002 - Mexico
Exposure to someone with a communicable disease? None

Drug or Food Allergy Or Sensitivity

Drug or Food Name	Reaction
Penicillin	Rash on body
Peanuts	Difficulty breathing

Current Medication

Medication Name	Dosage	Times per Day	Last Dose Taken
Digoxin	0.25 mg	Daily	9 am
Apresoline	50 mg	Twice	9 am
Aspirin	81 mg	Daily	9 am
Milk of Magnesia	1 ounce	When needed	Last night

Describe the typical weekly routine for this person.

Activity Level: Walks 2 miles per day. Swims in the ocean 4 times per week.
Stress Level – stress level is low.
Work Setting – retired but volunteers as a docent.
Other factors the medical team should know – Lives by herself. Drives and is very independent. Has had two periods of dizziness in the past week.

The other half of "hospital readiness" is to have complete legal forms that should accompany the advocate and patient to the hospital. These include the Living Will and Medical Power of Attorney (sometimes called "Durable Power of Attorney for Health Care or "Advance Health Care Directive.") These two documents are known by the general term "Advance Directives," and refer to your oral and written instructions about your future medical care, in the event you become unable to speak for yourself. Each state regulates the use of advance directives differently. Advance directives give you a voice in decisions about your medical care when you are unconscious or too ill to communicate. As long as you are able to express your own decisions, your advance directives will not be used and you can accept or refuse any medical treatment. But if you become seriously ill, you may lose the ability to participate in decisions about your own treatment unless the physicians have your Advance Directives.

It is highly advisable that these documents be prepared before an individual becomes ill. While you can obtain these forms from your attorney, stationery store or from numerous Internet sites and complete them quickly, the patient may be too ill to give accurate information and/or understand what he or she is signing. Moreover, these documents often have to be notarized, which is much more difficult to accomplish if the patient has already been admitted to the hospital.

When making the decision for persons to represent you in legal matters, it is best to consult with an attorney. Your decision of who should represent you if you are unable to represent yourself must be carefully made. At times it might be best that the designee chosen as Durable Power of Attorney for Healthcare may not be a family member. For example, I am the Durable Power of Attorney for Healthcare for some of my friends, because they believe that their family members will be too emotionally involved and may not have the medical knowledge to make the best decision at the time.

Medical Power of Attorney

The following is the first page of a California Advance Healthcare Directive. It provides an explanation of the various sections of the document and what powers will be granted to whomever the patient designates. This document is typical of what most states require.

California Advance Healthcare Directive
(California Probate Code Section 4701)

Explanation: You have the right to give instructions about your own healthcare. You also have the right to name someone else to make healthcare decisions for you. This form lets you do either or both of these things. It also lets you express your wishes regarding donation of organs and the designation of your primary physician. If you use this form, you may complete or modify all or any part of it. You are free to use a different form.

Part 1 of this form is a Power of Attorney for Healthcare. Part 1 lets you name another individual as agent to make healthcare decisions for you if you become incapable of making your own decisions, or if you want someone else to make those decisions for you now even though you are still capable. You may also name an alternate agent to act for you if your first choice is not willing, able, or reasonably available to make decisions for you. (Your agent may not be an operator or employee of a community care facility or a residential care facility where you are receiving care, or your supervising healthcare provider or employee of the healthcare institution where you are receiving care, unless your agent is related to you or is a co-worker.)

Unless the form you sign limits the authority of your agent, your agent may make all healthcare decisions for you. This form has a place for you to limit the authority of your agent. You need not limit the authority of your agent if you wish to rely on your agent for all healthcare decisions that may have to be made. If you choose not to limit the authority of your agent, your agent will have the right to:

a. Consent or refuse consent to any care, treatment, service, or procedure to maintain, diagnose, or otherwise affect a physical or mental condition.

b. Select or discharge healthcare providers and institutions.

c. Approve or disapprove diagnostic tests, surgical procedures, and programs of medication.

d. Direct the provision, withholding, or withdrawal of artificial nutrition and hydration and all other forms of healthcare, including cardiopulmonary resuscitation.

e. Make anatomical gifts, authorize an autopsy, and direct disposition of remains.

Part 2 of this form lets you give specific instructions about any aspect of your healthcare, whether or not you appoint an agent. Choices are provided for you to express your wishes regarding the provision, withholding, or withdrawal of treatment to keep you alive, as well as the provision of pain relief. Space is also provided for you to add to the choices you have made or for you to write out any additional wishes. If you are satisfied to allow your agent to determine what is best for you in making end-of-life decisions, you need not fill out Part 2 of this form.

Part 3 of this form lets you express an intention to donate your bodily organs and tissues following your death.

Part 4 of this form lets you designate a physician to have primary responsibility for your healthcare.

After completing this form, sign and date the form at the end. The form must be signed by two qualified witnesses or acknowledged before a notary public. Give a copy of the signed and completed form to your physician, to any other healthcare providers you may have, to any healthcare institution at which you are receiving care, and to any healthcare agents you have named. You should talk to the person you have named as agent to make sure that he or she understands your wishes and is willing to take the responsibility. You have the right to revoke this advance healthcare directive or replace this form at any time.

Living Will

The other part of Advanced Directives is the Living Will. The following is a sample of a Living Will. The form has been edited to show you the key components. Do not use this form as shown here. You will need to find a form that is appropriate to your state and your needs. The Website on the Internet where you can find information and forms can be found in the Reference Pages in the Appendix.

LIVING WILL OF_____

I, _____, a resident of the City of _____, _____ County, State of _____, being of sound and disposing mind, memory and understanding, do hereby willfully and voluntarily make, publish and declare this to be my LIVING WILL, making known my desire that my life shall not be artificially prolonged under the circumstances set forth below, and do hereby declare:

l. This instrument is directed to my family, my physician(s), my attorney, my clergyman, any medical facility in whose care I happen to be, and to any individual who may become responsible for my health, welfare or affairs.

2. Death is as much a reality as birth, growth, maturity and old age. It is the one certainty of life. Let this statement stand as an expression of my wishes now that I am still of sound mind, for the time when I may no longer take part in decisions for my own future.

3. If, at any time, I should have a terminal condition and my attending physician has determined that there can be no recovery from such condition and my death is imminent, where the application of life-prolonging procedures and "heroic measures" would serve only to artificially prolong the dying process, I direct that such procedures be withheld or withdrawn,

and that I be permitted to die naturally. I do not fear death itself as much as the indignities of deterioration, dependence and hopeless pain. I therefore ask that medication be mercifully administered to me and that any medical procedures be performed on me which are deemed necessary to provide me with comfort, care or to alleviate pain.

4. In the absence of my ability to give directions regarding the use of such life-prolonging procedures, it is my intention that this declaration shall be honored by my family and physician as the final expression of my legal right to refuse medical or surgical treatment and accept the consequences for such refusal.

5. In the event that I am diagnosed as comatose, incompetent, or otherwise mentally or physically incapable of communication, I appoint _____ to make binding decisions concerning my medical treatment.

6. If I have been diagnosed as pregnant and that diagnosis is known to my physician, this declaration shall have no force or effect during the course of my pregnancy.

7. I understand the full import of this declaration and I am emotionally and mentally competent to make this declaration. I hope you, who care for me, will feel morally bound to follow its mandate. I recognize that this appears to place a heavy responsibility upon you, but it is with the intention of relieving you of such responsibility and of placing it upon myself, in accordance with my strong convictions, that this statement is made.

While the Healthcare Directive and Living Will are binding legal documents, there are still many questions that surround the application of these documents. The following is a series of the most frequently asked questions about advanced directives and answers that hopefully should clarify the use of both of these forms.

1. WHAT IS A LIVING WILL?

A Living Will is a type of advance directive in which you put in writing your wishes about medical treatment should you be unable to communicate at the end of life. Your state law may define when the Living Will goes into effect, and may limit the treatments to which the Living Will applies. States name this document differently: for example it might be called a Directive to Physician, Declaration or Medical Directive. Your right to accept or refuse treatment is protected by constitutional and common law as well as state law.

2. WHAT IS A MEDICAL POWER OF ATTORNEY?

A Medical Power of Attorney is a document that lets you appoint someone you trust to make decisions about your medical care if you cannot make those decisions yourself. This type of advance directive also may be called a healthcare Proxy, Appointment of Healthcare Agent or a Durable Power of Attorney for Healthcare. The person you appoint through a Medical Power of Attorney normally is authorized to speak for you any time you are unable to make your own medical decisions, not only at the end of life.

3. WHO NEEDS TO PREPARE AN ADVANCE DIRECTIVE?

These are not just for the elderly. A serious accident could happen to anyone, so every adult over the age of 18 should prepare an Advance Directive. Several landmark legal cases dealing with the rights of individuals to refuse unwanted medical treatments have involved young people under the age of 30, including those dealing with Karen Ann Quinlan and Nancy Cruzan. The case involving Nancy Cruzan was heard by the United States Supreme Court.

4. DO I NEED BOTH A LIVING WILL AND A MEDICAL POWER OF ATTORNEY?

Yes, you can best protect your treatment wishes by having a Living Will and appointing a healthcare agent. Each offers something the other does not. The appointment of an agent ensures a more flexible form of decision-making, since the agent can respond to unanticipated changes and base decisions not only on written or verbal expressions of treatment wishes, but also on general knowledge of the patient. None the less, the Living Will can be very useful for several reasons.

If the agent becomes unavailable or unwilling to serve, the Living Will can serve to guide medical decision making. The Living Will can reassure the agent that he or she is following the wishes of the principal and ease the burden of decision-making. If the agent's decisions are challenged, the Living Will can provide evidence that the agent is acting in good faith. Finally, not everyone has someone to serve as a healthcare agent.

5. WHERE DO I GET THESE DOCUMENTS?

Your local hospital or long-term care facility may distribute them. Some physicians make them available to their patients. You can also get them for a nominal charge through Partnership for Caring by calling 800.989.9455. You can download them at no charge from the Internet.

6. WHAT DO I DO WITH MY DIRECTIVES AFTER THEY ARE SIGNED?

Make several photocopies of the completed documents. Keep the original in a safe but accessible place (not a safe deposit box). Give the copies to your agent, alternate agent, your doctor and anyone else who might be involved with your healthcare.

7. WILL MY ADVANCE DIRECTIVES BE HONORED IN ANOTHER STATE?

Many states' laws explicitly honor out-of-state directives as long as they do not conflict with that state's own law and other state statutes don't address the issue. In fact, a state would probably have to honor an Advance Directive that clearly expressed your treatment wishes, because your constitutional and common-law rights to accept or refuse treatment may be even broader than your rights under a specific state law. However, if you spend significant time in more than one state, we recommend that you complete the Advance Directives for all of the states involved. It will be easier to have your Advance Directives honored if they are the ones with which the medical facility is familiar.

8. WILL MY ADVANCE DIRECTIVES BE HONORED IN AN EMERGENCY?

No. Generally, Advance Directives such as Living Wills and Medical Powers of Attorney are not effective in a medical emergency. There is no time in an emergency either to consult the directions in an Advance Directive or determine a person's underlying medical condition. Once the person comes under the care of a physician, the contents of a Living Will can be evaluated and the instructions of a healthcare agent determined in light of that person's overall prognosis.

9. WHAT HAPPENS IF MY DOCTOR (OR FAMILY) WON'T HONOR MY WISHES?

There is no simple answer to this question. For this reason, it is essential that you have honest and open discussions with your agent, family members and physician about their willingness to support and if necessary, advocate to see that your wishes are carried out. If you find they are not willing to support your choices, you may wish to consider appointing a non-family member who will honor your wishes or change your physician before a conflict arises. If you wish to talk about this further, call Partnership for Caring at 800.989.9455.

10. IF I SIGN ADVANCE DIRECTIVES, WILL DOCTORS STILL TAKE CARE OF ME IF I'M SICK?

Yes, a doctor or hospital cannot condition treatment on whether or not you have an Advance Directive. Even if you decline certain kinds of treatment, you may need care to ensure that you are kept comfortable and free of pain.

Once you have Advance Directives, you may want to fill out a card like this and place it in your wallet. A blank card sample is in Appendix B.

Advance Directive Card

Name: Hilda Shaylor

I have an Advance Directive on File at:

555 Main Street, Anywhere USA 80000

Call my Attorney: John Doe at (555) 123-4567

In addition to the Advance Directives, another helpful tool to have prepared is a Durable Power of Attorney for Financial Matters. This document identifies who will make your financial decisions for you should you be unable to make them independently. The following is an example of this type of document. Again, this is only a sample that has been edited to show you the key components. Internet sites can be found in the Appendix.

Durable Power of Attorney for Financial Matters

CALIFORNIA GENERAL DURABLE POWER OF ATTORNEY
THE POWERS YOU GRANT BELOW ARE EFFECTIVE
ONLY IF YOU BECOME DISABLED OR INCOMPETENT.

Caution: a Durable Power of Attorney is an important legal document. By signing the Durable Power of Attorney, you are authorizing another person to act for you, the principal. Before you sign a Durable Power of Attorney, you should know these important facts: your agent (attorney-in-fact) has no duty to act unless you and your agent agree otherwise in writing. This document gives your agent the powers to manage, dispose of, sell, and convey your real and personal property, and to use your property as security if your agent borrows money on your behalf. This document does not give your agent the power to accept or receive any of your property, in trust or otherwise, as a gift, unless you specifically authorize the agent to accept or receive a gift. The powers you give your agent will continue to exist for your entire lifetime, unless you state that the Durable Power of Attorney will last for a shorter period of time or unless you otherwise terminate the Durable Power of Attorney.

The powers you give your agent in this Durable Power of Attorney will continue to exist even if you can no longer make your own decisions respecting the management of your property. You can amend or change this Durable Power of Attorney only by executing a new Durable Power of Attorney or by executing an amendment through the same formalities as an original. You have the right to revoke or terminate this Durable Power of Attorney at any time, so long as you are competent.

This Durable Power of Attorney must be dated and must be acknowledged before a notary public or signed by two witnesses. A Durable Power of Attorney that may affect real property should be acknowledged before a notary public so that it may easily be recorded.

You should read the Durable Power of Attorney carefully. When effective, the Durable Power of Attorney will give your agent the right to deal with property that you now have or might acquire in the future. The Durable Power of Attorney is important to you. If you do not understand the Durable Power of Attorney, or any provision of it, then you should obtain the assistance of an attorney or other qualified person.

Notice to person accepting the appointment as attorney-in-fact by acting or agreeing to act as the agent (attorney-in-fact) under this Power of Attorney. You assume the fiduciary and other legal responsibilities of an agent. These responsibilities include:

1. The legal duty to act solely in the interest of the principal and to avoid conflicts of interest.

2. The legal duty to keep the principal's property separate and distinct from any other property owned or controlled by

you. You may not transfer the principal's property to yourself without full and adequate consideration or accept a gift of the principal's property unless this Power of Attorney specifically authorizes you to transfer property to yourself or accept a gift of the principal's property. If you transfer the principal's property to yourself without specific authorization in the Power of Attorney, you may be prosecuted for fraud and/or embezzlement. If the principal is 65 years of age or older at the time that the property is transferred to you without authority, you may also be prosecuted for elder abuse under penal code section 368. In addition to criminal prosecution, you may also be sued in civil court. I have read the foregoing notice and I understand the legal and fiduciary duties that I assume by acting or agreeing to act as the agent (attorney-in-fact) under the terms of this Power of Attorney.

Other legal forms may be helpful to have in place prior to someone becoming ill. An attorney can be very helpful in advising the most appropriate tools. Planning ahead for financial concerns such as a Living Trust may also be beneficial in planning for the future.

Bedside Story

Hilda was in a hospital that provided training for many medical students. She was assessed, reassessed and asked the same thing over and over. Many times when I was there, I would give the health team a summary of her health history. This allowed her to conserve her energy and helped her rest. The health team seemed appreciative of the information that I provided. There were also times when Hilda was confused and could not have given accurate information.

With Hilda, we used and updated the items in the Durable Power of Attorney forms on a regular basis. Hilda had indicated to us that she definitely did not want to be on life support. At the hospital, the physician orders included life support if necessary. We spoke with the physician, who was reluctant to change the order. He stated that he had talked with Hilda and she thought life support would "be all right." This was done while Hilda's lab values were abnormal, and she was slightly confused. When the physician refused to change the order, I insisted writing on the chart that Hilda had verbalized to her family and others on numerous occasions that she did not want life support should there need to be a decision. I emphasized that I was her Durable Power of Attorney for healthcare and was making this decision for her. I indicated that her family desired that her wishes be met. After the note was placed on the chart, the order was changed.

In order to communicate most effectively, I think it would be helpful to have written information readily available to give to those who come into the room. The hospital where Hilda stayed had a white board in each room. We readily used the white board to remind ourselves of information and requests we wanted to convey to the medical team. If there is no white board in the room, I would recommend buying some sheet of erasable white board from a office supply store and putting it in the patient's room.

*Key Points

- Develop a database for the patient that is kept with the patient and yourself.

- Update the database as conditions change.

- Have legal forms completed, before someone you love becomes ill.

- Consult an attorney, if necessary, before making legal decisions.

- Communicate regularly with the healthcare team about the wishes of the patient.

- Have one physician who can be the main contact for the patient to help put the puzzle together for the family to help them make informed decisions.

Who, What and Where in the Hospital

It's so confusing, who to ask,
Which nurse or doctor does what task.
One specializes in the brain,
While others deal in breaks and sprains.

The hospitals, they too confound,
As many services abound.
Department staffs should do their best
To put your many fears to rest.

So be assertive, ask the who
And when and where and what to do.
The expertise is always there,
You'll be surprised, how much they care.

CHAPTER 3
Who, What and Where in the Hospital

For most people, a hospital is a maze of corridors, offices, rooms, and waiting areas. Some doors are to be opened by "Authorized Personnel Only". Other doors are marked with signs indicating medical specialties or the name of an office.

In an effort to keep informed about the treatment a patient is receiving, advocates often need to ask questions and/or find out additional information that is located within the hospital. The following is a list of services and units, identified by their function or area of expertise. The list should provide guidance for an advocate seeking clarification, answers, and help.

Service	Function
Admissions Department	Handles admission process and necessary paperwork. May assist with routing the patient for the proper lab and x-ray exams.
Business Office	Handles insurance and financial affairs upon discharge.
Dialysis	For patients who have had failure of the kidneys and need their blood filtered.
Dietary or Nutritional Services	Supervises food preparation and helps choose the correct foods for a given diet.
ECG/EKG- electrocardiogram	Records electrical activity of the heart to determine heart rhythm, heart attack, heart chamber size and other abnormalities.
EEG- Electro-encephalography	Records brain waves and helps determine electrical activity of the brain.
EMG – electromyogram	Records electrical activity in body muscles.

Service	Function
Home Care	Helps coordinate care that will be needed when the patient goes home.
Hospice	Provides care for dying patients and their families. May be a freestanding unit or may help with care at home.
Housekeeping	Maintains the cleanliness of the hospital environment.
Laboratory	Examines specimens such as tissues, feces, urine, amniotic fluid and spinal fluid.
Medical Records or Health Information	Maintains and stores all medical records. This is the area where you may make a request to get copies of your own records.
Nursing Units	Provision of Basic Nursing Care. Staffed by a unit secretary, R.N.s, LVNs/LPNs and Nurses' Aides.
Occupational Therapy	Works with clients who have functional impairment to teach basic skills, such as grooming, feeding, dressing and bathing (activities of daily living).
Outpatient Surgery	Provides care to patients before and after same day surgery.
Pharmacy	Mixes and dispenses medications to the various units.
Physical Therapy	Works with patients with muscular and skeletal problems, assess strength and mobility, and performs therapeutic measures such as range of motion, massage, heat and cold; are responsible for teaching new skills such as crutch-walking.
Radiology (X-ray)	Includes standard x-rays as well as CT scans, MRI, mammography, ultrasound, arteriograms, venograms, and echocardiograms.
Respiratory Therapy	Provides breathing treatments, monitors ventilators, draws and analyzes arterial blood gases, performs pulmonary function testing. May be involved in taking EKGs.
Sleep Center	Provides observation, testing and monitoring of patients while they sleep. Often done to diagnose sleep apnea.

Service	Function
Social Services	Helps patients with psychosocial problems to provide assistance with housing, finances, and referral to support groups; is often the person to help with abuse reporting.
Speech Therapy	Assists patients with speech impairments to speak understandably or to learn other methods of communication.
Spiritual Needs	Some facilities have a resident chaplain, but all facilities can provide support for almost any religion by making a phone call. The nursing supervisor may be a good resource to help with this.
Nursing Areas	**Function**
(CCU) Coronary Care Unit	Provides care to patients with heart attack or heart surgery.
(ICU) Intensive Care Unit	Provides care to critically ill patients.
DOU– Definitive Observation Unit	Serves patients who need cardiac monitoring. Often, patients are transferred from ICU or CCU to this area.
Emergency Department	Provides care for patients involved in accidents and medical emergencies.
Medical Unit	For patients with medical problems, such as diabetes and congestive heart failure.
Mental Health Unit	Serves patients who have had difficulty with relationships, coping, or are in crisis.
Orthopedic Unit	Serves patients who have had fractures or broken bones.
Psychiatric Unit	Serves clients diagnosed as having a mental illness.
Rehabilitation	Provides care for patients who must regain the highest level of self-care following injury, accident, or illness, such as spinal cord injury or stroke.
Surgical Unit	Serves patients who have recently undergone surgery.
Transitional Care Unit	Cares for patients transitioning from the acute nursing unit to convalescent care or possible hospital discharge.

The Medical Team

The medical team that serves an individual patient consists of many persons with talents and skills that are unique and distinct. Team members include nurses, physicians, therapists, and others that are called in to meet the particular needs of a patient. The team member who is most knowledgeable about all aspects of the patient and coordinates care is the registered nurse (RN) who serves as the case manager. The case manager works closely with a general practitioner or internist, who directs which specialists will be needed to serve the patient. The case manager facilitates communication among the physicians, ensures that needed services and ongoing care are provided, prevents the duplication of services, is responsible for assessment, and spends the most hours with the patient.

The following charts provide identifying information about possible members of the medical team, along with their credentials, roles, and responsibilities, as well as physicians and their specialties. An additional list of physicians and their specialties are in the Appendix.

HEALTH TEAM MEMBERS

Team Member	Education	Role
Case Manager-usually a Registered Nurse	2 – 4 years of college. From Associate degree to a Master's degree.	Tracks patient progress through the health system to ensure continuity; helps with coordination of care in the hospital and discharge.
Licensed Vocational Nurse (LVN), Licensed Practical Nurse (LPN)	1 to 1 ½ years of vocational training.	Assists in patient care; administers treatments and I.V. fluids; administers medications, but generally I.V. meds; works under the direction of an R.N.

Team Member	Education	Role
Nursing Assistant (NA), Certified Nursing (CNA)	6 weeks to 6 months of vocational training.	Performs basic care such as vital signs, beds and baths; can assist in activities of daily living (feeding, oral hygiene, ROM, basic activity); does not administer medications in most states.
Registered Nurse (RN)	2 – 4 years of college.	Plans care; implements physician's orders; coordinates care on the unit; performs treatments; administers medications and I.V.s.
Occupational Therapist (OT)	4 years of college	Works with patient to help with activities of daily living such as grooming, dressing, feeding, transferring and bathing.
Physical Therapist (PT), Licensed Physical Therapist (LPT)	4+ years of college	Works with clients with musculoskeletal disorders; assists with range of motion, massage, whirlpool, heat and cold, crutch walking, mobility and transfers.
Physician or Doctor of Osteopathy (DO)	8+ years of college	Formulates medical diagnosis; administers procedures and directs care via orders; also has training in muscle and bone manipulation.
Physician or Medical Doctor (MD)	8+ years of college	Formulates medical diagnosis; administers procedures; directs care via orders
Physician Assistant (PA)	4 – 6 years of college	Provides medical services under the supervision of a physician.
Psychiatric Technician (PT)	1 to 1 ½ years of vocational training.	Provides care to patients with mental disorders or developmental disabilities; performs treatments and administers medications, but not I.V.s.; primarily in California.
Registered Dietician (RD)	4+ years of college	Plans nutritional needs of the patient; calculates metabolic rate and correlates lab data to determine special dietary needs to help the patient.

Team Member	Education	Role
Registered Pharmacist (RPh)	5 – 6 years of college	Prepares and dispenses drugs; educates patients about their medications.
Respiratory Therapist (RT), Respiratory Care Practitioner (RCP), Certified Respiratory Therapy Tech. (CRTT)	2 – 4 years of college	Administers pulmonary function tests; performs breathing treatments; oversees care for ventilator and oxygen administration; draws and analyzes arterial blood gases.
Social Worker (SW), Master's of Social Work (MSW)	4 – 6 years of college	Assists clients with psycho-social problems, such as financial, housing, and personal.
Speech Therapist	4 years of college	Helps patients with speech impairments to speak clearly or to learn other methods of communication; may also work with swallowing difficulties.
Spiritual Help	Varied- up to 8 years of college or training	Assists in meeting spiritual needs; provides counseling and family support and conducts religious services.

PHYSICIANS

Specialist	Area of Responsibility
Anesthesiologist	Delivers anesthesia during surgery to provide pain relief.
Cardiologist	Treats heart and vascular disorders.
Endocrinologist	Treats endocrine gland disorders, including diabetes and thyroid.
Family Practitioner	Treats children and adults on a continuing basis; provides a referral base for other specialties.
Gastroenterologist	Treats disorders of the stomach, intestines, gallbladder and bile duct.

Specialist	Area of Responsibility
Gynecologist	Treats the female reproductive system.
Hospitalist	Hospitalists are physicians who spend at least 25 percent of their professional time serving as the physicians-of-record for inpatients. They return the patients back to the care of their primary care providers at the time of hospital discharge.
Internist	Provides non-surgical treatment for adult disorders.
Neurologist	Provides non-surgical treatment for disorders of the nervous system.
Oncologist	Treats various forms of cancer.
Pulmonologist	Provides treatment for lung and breathing disorders.
Radiologist	Takes and reads x-rays to diagnose and treat disorders.
Urologist	Treats the male urinary and reproductive systems and the female urinary system.

A major role that an advocate can play in working with the medical team is that of a liaison among the many specialists who will be in to treat the patient. That number can be compounded in a teaching institution where four persons in one specialty such as an intern, resident, fellow, and attending physician may come to the bedside to ask questions, assess, and make notations on the chart. These specialists tend to concentrate on one body part and are reluctant to field questions or treat other body parts.

Do not assume that the medical team is closely communicating with each other. The medical team rarely meets together, and although all consultations and treatments are documented in the chart, one doctor rarely reads all of the other doctors' notes.

One team member who can be very helpful in coordinating care and communicating with the various team players is the case manager. The case manager is most often a registered nurse who is overseeing care, often with the goal of getting the patient discharged as soon as safely possible. If the facility has a case management process, ask to see the case manager assigned to the patient. The case manager is often a resourceful, helpful person who can help you in frustrating situations.

Tips for working with the medical team:

Once the members of the patient's medical team have been determined and identified, the advocate can actively contribute to the care of the patient by cooperating with the team and engaging in any/some/all of the following activities:

- Be the liaison. The patient is often too fatigued or disoriented to repeat the same story to so many persons or keep track of who has come and gone.

- Inform the healthcare team that you are advocating for the patient.

- Introduce yourself to team members and find out who they are and what they do.

- Take notes on every event and conversation that occurs between the nurse and/or doctor and patient. This is especially important because you as the advocate may need to provide a history of what has recently happened. Sometimes doctors are unaware of medication changes or changes in the patient's condition. Because doctors often do not thoroughly read the patient's chart, they miss important information that other physicians and nurses have recorded. The advocate can be invaluable as a communicator of vital information to the medical staff.

- Watch to see that team members are washing their hands prior to touching the patient.

- Try to become knowledgeable about impending treatments. If an upcoming treatment requires that the patient is to take nothing by mouth for a number of hours prior to the test, be sure nobody offers food or fluids.

- Be aware of the patient's food and medication allergies. Check the meal trays to be sure that those foods that will cause adverse effects are not being served. If new medications are ordered, use the Internet or medication reference books to be sure that the new drugs are not related to drugs that the patient cannot safely take, make sure that the new medication will not interact adversely with medications the patient is already taking.

- Work closely with the case manager; because of her role as overseer of the patient's care with the goal of getting the patient discharged as soon as it is safely possible, the case manager has many resources at his/her disposal.

- Ask questions, be assertive, and intervene when necessary on behalf of the patient.

As stated earlier, the medical team seldom meets as a group. While each doctor who visits a patient places notations and instructions on the chart, there is no guarantee that doctors will even read or pay attention to what other physicians have written.

You can help by knowing who is participating in the care of your loved one. Ask questions of all the practitioners. Ask them what their roles are and if you can provide any needed information. Read your daily logs and follow through to see that requests have been honored. Consider yourself an integral part of the medical team.

Here is a tool that may help you communicate with the medical team as they see the patient. Blank forms can be found in Appendix D.

Communication Log

Patient Name <u>Hilda Shaylor</u> Lead Advocate <u>Terry Rudd</u>
Other Advocate <u>Linda Cooper or Trish Billings</u>
Allergies <u>Penicillin, Peanuts</u>

Physicians to See Patient

Physician	Specialty	Date Seen	Communication
Dr. Patel	Cardiology	Feb. 2	Said that Mom's heart rhythm had changed and would need medication to stabilize.
Dr. Chin	Gastroenterology	Feb 3	Said that Mom may have an ulcer and will be started on a medication in the IV to help prevent ulcers.

Other Persons to See Patient

Person	Specialty	Date Seen	Communication
May Lee	Dietician	2/3	Said the protein was low and needs to eat foods high in protein.
John Brown	Physical Therapy	2/4	Said that mom isn't exercising enough. Said she can do her upper body herself, but will need help with the lower body.

Patient Complaints

Date	Concern	Person Notified	Communication	Date Resolved
2/3	Food is Bland	Nurse – Nancy	Asked to have someone from dietary talk to mom about better- tasting food	
2/4	Has a cough	Nurse – Michael	Mom has a cough and a tickle in her throat. Mike will notify the doctor	2/4 pm – breathing treatment

Advocate Concerns

Date	Concern	Person Notified	Communication	Date Resolved
2/3	Only ate 25% of food	Nurse – Nancy	Waiting for dietary to come up to talk to patient	
2/4	Internist has not seen her for 2 days	Nurse – Michael	I am worried about her blood pressure	
2/5	Patient in next bed is coughing a lot	Nurse – Mary	Waiting to talk to nurse	

Communication is essential. The initial tools given in Chapter 2 are helpful for recording the medical history. Keeping communication logs lets the medical team know your overall concerns and gives you a method to track questions, problems and their resolutions.

Bedside Story

At one point in time, Hilda had 18 different physicians seeing her in one day. This did not include the nurses, therapists, and ancillary staff. We joked that only a pediatrician, gynecologist and podiatrist failed to attend! Our family found that our knowledge of what was happening with Hilda's care superceded that of any individual team member. I found I was frequently repeating to the next person entering the room what had happened before. Often, the practitioner was unaware of a change in condition or medication that had been initiated. There were a number of occasions where we prevented an error from occurring by communicating to a team member that a procedure or treatment had been done or terminated for a specific reason.

*Key Points

- Know who's who on the healthcare team.
- Consider yourself a member of the medical team.
- Keep communication logs and let the medical team know your concerns.
- Follow through to make sure requests have been honored.

Notes

_____

_____

_____

_____

_____

_____

_____

_____

_____

_____

_____

_____

_____

_____

_____

_____

_____

_____

_____

_____

Interpreting Medical Abbreviations and Terms

When doctors talk to other staff
A layman might have cause to laugh;
Our ignorance do not malign,
Interpreters should be assigned.

'Cause P.O. does not mean you're mad,
And C.H.F. is really bad;
When CAD is not a man to hate,
And BUN is not some bread you ate.

This jargon gives us cause to muse
Because it masks so many clues
So research, read, and ask away;
Your vigilance may save the day.

CHAPTER 4
Interpreting Medical Abbreviations And Terms

Every profession develops its own language that is not easily understood by those without training in that field. The written and oral communication among doctors, nurses and other staff is usually conducted using abbreviations and acronyms because it saves time when talking and space when writing on a chart. The patient or advocate needs to understand what is being said or written in order to follow and monitor the care that is being prescribed. Learning medical terminology can help the family "get a handle" on what medical personnel are talking about.

The following chart provides translations and explanations for the most commonly used abbreviations, acronyms, and terms used by doctors and members of the medical team. Additional abbreviations can be found in the Appendix.

Summary of Common Medical Abbreviations

ABBREVIATION	MEANING
ABG	Arterial blood gas Measures levels, especially oxygen in the arterial blood.
a.c.	Before meals
ADL	Activities of daily living Includes bathing, grooming, eating and teeth brushing.
Afib	Atrial fibrillation – a heart rhythm abnormality.

ABBREVIATION	MEANING
b.i.d.	Twice a day. Used in the timing of treatments and medications.
BP	Blood pressure. One of the vital signs.
BUN	Blood urea nitrogen. A blood test usually to determine functioning of the kidneys.
c*	With. A shorthand notation. *There is a line drawn above this abbreviation.
CA, Ca, ca	Cancer, carcinoma, calcium. Because of its multiple uses, the context of how the term is used will determine its meaning.
CABG	Coronary artery bypass graft. Open heart surgery to bypass blockage of the coronary arteries.
CBC	Complete blood count. A blood test to determine if a person is anemic.
CC, C.C., cc	Chief complaint is the main reason the person came in the hospital. A cubic centimeter is the same as a milliliter, a small liquid measure.
CHF	Congestive heart failure. A common heart condition where the heart muscle is too weak to handle the blood volume.
COPD	Chronic obstructive pulmonary disease. A general term that can include asthma, emphysema or bronchitis.
CPK or CK	Creatine phosphokinase. An enzyme level to check for damage to the heart muscle and to diagnose a heart attack.
C&S	Culture and sensitivity. Blood test to identify bacteria (culture) and determine which antibiotic is most useful for that bacteria (sensitivity).
CT, CAT Scan	Computed tomography, computerized axial tomography. An x-ray exam used for identifying tumors, bleeding, or structural abnormalities.
CVA	Cerebrovascular accident. Also called a stroke or a brain attack. Caused by a disruption of the blood flow to the brain.

ABBREVIATION	MEANING
DC	Discharge or discontinue.
DM	Diabetes mellitus. A disorder of metabolism of substances into the cell from a lack of insulin.
DX, Dx, dx	Diagnosis abbreviation.
ECG, EKG	Electrocardiogram. A test to check the electrical activity of the heart. An EKG can identify heart rhythm and may be helpful in diagnosing a heart attack.
ED, ER	Emergency department or room.
FBS	Fasting blood sugar. A blood sugar or blood glucose test. May require up to 12 hours of fasting.
Fx	Fracture
g, gm	Gram. A unit of measure. Most drugs are given in milligrams or grams.
Hb, Hgb	Hemoglobin. Part of the complete blood count. Determines oxygen carrying capacity of the blood.
HCT	Hematocrit. Part of the complete blood count that helps measure hydration and anemias.
HR	Heart rate. Same as the pulse. The normal range is 60-100 beats per minute. Children and infants have higher normal rates.
Hr, H	Hour
h.s.	At bedtime, hour of sleep. Some medications are given at hour of sleep.
Hx	History. An abbreviation to determine the patient's medical and social history.
ICU	Intensive care unit. An area in the hospital for patients who are critically ill.
I.M.	Intramuscular. A method of giving an injection that goes deep into the muscle.

ABBREVIATION	MEANING
I&O	Intake and output. Patients are often on I & O. Everything that the patient takes in such as fluid and food is measured. Also, whatever is put out, such as urine, stool, and drainage is also measured. If your family member is on I & O, it is very important that you let the nursing staff know what has been taken in. Be careful not to flush the toilet as that output also needs to be measured.
K	Potassium. The symbol for the blood test to check this value.
KO or KVO	Keep open. A term used for the intravenous fluid that is running at a very low rate just to keep the vein open.
mEq	Milliequivalent. Substances such as potassium are measured in mEq.
Mg	Magnesium. A substance in the body.
mg	Milligram. A unit of measure used to determine drug amounts.
M.I.	Myocardial infarction. Heart attack.
ml	Milliliter. A liquid unit of measure.
MRI	Magnetic resonance imaging. A radiology exam used for locating tumors, structural abnormalities and bleeding.
MS	Multiple sclerosis, morphine sulfate
Na	Sodium. An electrolyte in the body. A common blood test.
NGT, NG	Nasogastric tube. A tube passed from the nose into the stomach to either give feedings or remove fluids from the stomach.
NKA	No known allergies.
NPO	Nothing (can be taken) by mouth. If the person is NPO, make sure you do not offer food or fluids.
N.S.	Normal saline. Salt water solution.

ABBREVIATION	MEANING
P	Phosphorus, pulse. Pulse is the same as heart rate with a range of 60-100 beats per minute. P with a line over it is after.
p.c.	After meals. Some medications are given p.c. for better absorption.
P.O.	By mouth.
p.r.n.	As needed, whenever necessary. When a medication or treatment is ordered PRN the patient needs to ask for the item. Pain medications, laxatives, and sleeping pills are often ordered PRN.
Pro time, PT	Prothrombin time. A blood test to measure the effect of the drug Warfarin (Coumadin). When the patient is on this drug, the pro time should be prolonged above normal range.
PT	Physical therapy, Psychiatric Technician, Patient, pint
q	Every.
q.d.	Every day
q.h.	Every hour
q2h, q4h	Every 2 hours, Every 4 hours
q.i.d.	Four times a day
R	Respirations. The number of breaths per minute. The range is 12-20 per minute.
RBC	Red blood cell. Part of the complete blood count. Determines oxygen carrying capacity and to determine anemia.
RN	Registered nurse. This person is the person who is responsible for the day-to-day care. There is almost always an RN working on each unit.
R/O	Rule out. This term is used when the team is working on the actual diagnosis.
ROM	Range of motion (of joint). Exercises given to help with joint movement and muscle tone. Ask the staff if you can participate in helping with ROM.

ABBREVIATION	MEANING
Rx	Prescription
S.C., SQ, subq	Subcutaneous. A method for giving an injection.
SOB	Short of breath (Yes, this is really an abbreviation)
S&S	Signs and symptoms
stat	Immediately. Used for treatment or medication to be given right away.
Sx	Symptom
TB	Tuberculosis
T&C	Type and cross match. Test of the blood for type and matching potential prior to getting a transfusion.
temp., T	Temperature. The normal range for oral temperature is 97.6 – 99.6 degrees Fahrenheit or 36.5 – 37 Celsius.
t.i.d.	Three times a day
TPR	Temperature, pulse, respirations. Three of the vital signs.
Tx	Treatment
UA	Urinalysis. Urine test to determine presence of bacteria or an alteration.
VS	Vital signs. Includes temperature, pulse, respiration, blood pressure, and pain assessment.
WBC	White blood cell. The number, measured through a blood test, indicates the severity of an infection.

The patient or advocate needs to understand what is being said or written in order to follow and monitor the care that is being prescribed. Once the jargon becomes decipherable, he or she can ask more intelligent, informed questions about the patient's condition. Also, remember that if you are an advocate with a Durable Power of Attorney for Healthcare, you have the right to look at the patient's chart and take as many notes as you need to in order to find what is going on. Ask for help if you cannot read the doctors' handwriting. Purchasing a paperback medical terminology book or spending time on the Internet is a good idea and will help you more thoroughly understand the patient's condition.

Bedside Story

The medical terminology, for me, was generally not a problem, but I soon realized I needed to be the interpreter for everyone who visited her. There were also times when I needed to ask the medical team to define a term or concept for me, and even though Hilda had been a Registered Nurse, there were many times I needed to explain concepts and terms to her.

*Key Points

- Have medical terminology resources close at hand.
- Ask questions if you don't understand.
- Ask your loved one if they have any questions and help them with explanations and definitions.

Notes

_____

_____

_____

_____

_____

_____

_____

_____

_____

_____

_____

Notes

Measuring Vital Signs

Your temperature, they'll take for sure,
As part of looking for a cure.
While 98.6 sounds swell,
A 37 works as well.

Yet other vital signs can lend
Some hints on just how fast you'll mend.
A respiration check will show
Your breathing rate- too fast or slow?

Blood pressure, and the pain you feel,
Along with pulse will help reveal
The values that the doctors need,
To tell them how they should proceed

CHAPTER 5
Measuring Vital Signs

Vital signs are the basic measures that are used to find out if the body is giving us a message about something being ill or injured. The five basic vital signs are temperature, pulse, respiration, blood pressure and pain. Vital signs are taken on admission to a particular medical unit and at various intervals, depending upon the condition of the patient.

General guidelines for the timing and occurrence of vital signs are listed below:

- On admission to a unit
- At the beginning of each shift
- One or more times during an 8 hour nursing shift
- Two more times during a 12 hour nursing shift
- Prior to the administration of medications that may affect heart rate or blood pressure
- After surgery – every 15 minutes for the first hour.
- In intensive care units – usually hourly, but may be every 15 minutes, depending upon the patient's condition or physician's orders. As the patient becomes more stable, vital signs may be done every 2 hours and then every 4 hours.

The taking of vital signs does vary depending upon the need to check values. Do not be alarmed if vital signs are taken frequently. There may be variables that you are not aware of, such as a student needing to be double checked by an instructor, the medical team not realizing that the vitals had just been checked, or a possible change in condition. Many facilities monitor vital signs electronically in a way that allows you to see what the value reads. A patient or advocate may ask, at any time, what the patient's vital signs are.

Temperature

The temperature is usually measured to see if there is a fever, usually caused by infection or dehydration. A patient's temperature is taken by various means, depending upon his/her age, condition, and available equipment. Usually, the patient's temperature is taken by one of the following:

Oral – (Mouth)   Time period- 3 minutes
        Normal range: 97.6 - 99.6 degrees
Rectal – (Anus)   Time period- 3 minutes
        Normal range: 98.6 - 100.6 degrees
Axillary – (Armpit)   Time period- 10 minutes
        Normal range: 96.6 - 98.6
Otic or Tympanic   Time period- 10 seconds or less
        Normal range: is calibrated by the machine to oral or rectal normal readings.

In critical care units, body temperature is sometimes measured by a probe that is left in the rectum or by equipment that can calculate temperature from a urinary catheter. In these situations, you will not see the temperature taken by the methods listed above. Some factors that may affect a patient's temperature include smoking, drinking fluids or eating food right before the temperature is taken, and using oxygen.

Pulse

Another vital sign is the pulse, an indicator of how well the heart is functioning. The pulse is taken to measure both number of beats per minute, and rhythm, the regularity of the beats.

To measure the pulse rate, the number of beats is counted over a thirty second period. That number is then multiplied by two. The normal range for adults is 60 to 100 beats per minute. The optimal finding would be a strong and regular 80 per minute beat.

There are many ways that the pulse may be checked. The most common method is to check the radial pulse which is found on the inside of the wrist along the thumb line.

Other pulse sites include the following:

Temporal: Can be felt on temple, side of head
Carotid: On the neck on either side of the throat
Femoral: In the crease of the groin area
Pedal: On top of the foot (by the shoelaces)
Brachial: Inside of elbow

Other ways to check heart rate are by listening to the heart with a stethoscope, via heart monitor, or by a device called a Doppler, which provides the practitioner with an audible tone for the pulse.

Heart rates increase when the heart tries to get more oxygenated blood to the body tissues. Common causes of this reaction include stress, fever, increased activity, difficulty breathing and taking certain medications.

Heart rates tend to decrease from the effects of medication, straining, and disturbances in the conduction system of the heart.

Respirations

Measuring respirations indicates how many breaths per minute the patient is taking and is one of the most difficult vital signs to check. Each inhalation and exhalation equals one breath.

To measure respirations, the practitioner has to count the number of breaths a patient takes over a thirty second period and multiply that number by two. Adult patient breaths should measure between 12 to 20. Infant respirations are slightly higher, falling between 20 and 40. While measuring respirations, it is also important to monitor the rhythm, rate, depth and quality of each breath. Sensors on the cardiac monitor and on the ventilator may also be utilized to count respirations.

Respirations increase when the body attempts to get more oxygen to the body tissues. Respirations may decrease as the result of certain medications, especially narcotics.

Blood Pressure

Blood pressure is measured to determine how much pressure there is against the walls of the arteries. Blood pressure may be measured by a variety of methods including the standard cuff, electronic devices, and with a catheter placed directly into an artery.

Blood pressure is described by two numbers- a top number that measures pressure while the heart is contracting and a lower number that measures pressure while the heart is at rest. The top number is called the systolic pressure and ranges from 90 to 140. The bottom or lower number is the diastolic pressure and ranges from 60 to 90.

Hypertension or high blood pressure, is a reading that is above 140 systolic or over 90 diastolic. The long-term effects of hypertension can lead to a heart attack, congestive heart failure, stroke or failure of organs. While the cause of hypertension is unknown, stress, fluid retention and increased intake of salt are unwelcome conditions that may contribute to the condition.

Hypotension, or low blood pressure, can also be very dangerous. If the blood pressure is too low, the body may not be able to get blood to tissues. Organs and body systems, especially the kidneys, may fail. Low blood pressure may be caused by dehydration, blood loss, or certain medications.

Pain

Of all the vital signs, the most difficult to measure is pain, because there is no definitive value or scale, and each individual has a pain threshold that is unique.

Addressing, assessing and adequate treatment of pain is a priority, and all facilities use some type of pain scale. Some hospitals employ a 0-10 numerical scale, and the patient is asked to identify at what level the pain is that he/she is experiencing. Other hospitals use a series of pictures and ask patients to identify with one of the pictures.

Advocates should be aware that there are many techniques and medications that may help to alleviate pain, depending upon its cause and type.

Bedside Story

Hilda had a chronic condition called Atrial Fibrillation, which makes the pulse rhythm irregular. Since I knew this, I was able to communicate to members of the medical team who came into the room, that as a baseline, her pulse was irregular. I always kept a close watch on Hilda's vital signs, because they are the first indicators of problems and/or complications.

*Key Points

- Vital signs are the base measure to determine what may be wrong.

- Keep an eye on vital sign trends to see if there are changes.

- Question changes in vital signs and what may be happening. If the person you speak with doesn't have the answers, ask someone else.

- All patients have a right to have their pain assessed and treated appropriately. If pain concerns are not being met, talk to the nursing manager to see what may be done to help get better pain control.

Notes

Lab Tests and Diagnostic Procedures

A hospital one can attest,
Is not a place where one can rest.
Procedures and exams are musts,
So treatments doctors can adjust.

So cultures, blood and urine, too,
Are sent to labs for their review.
And many x-rays they will need,
Of organs that could ache or bleed.

And tubes inserted up or down
In those who wear hospital gowns.
Despite discomfort, tests will tell,
What doctors need to make you well.

Tests are the chief means by which physicians make their diagnoses. Certainly the untrained person cannot possibly understand all the nuances and implications of the results of diagnostic tests and procedures. However, it is possible for patients or advocates to understand enough about test results to ask informed, intelligent questions. The following charts will provide you with information about the most commonly ordered lab tests, diagnostic procedures and what you might ask or do with this information. Additional lab values and information can be found in Appendix F.

Remember to ask the physician if you don't understand the results or significance of a lab test or procedure. Initial results are often a guideline and may or may not mean the patient has that condition. Other tests will be administered to confirm a diagnosis.

Some abbreviations related to lab values include the following:

Mg	=	milligram
Mcg	=	microgram
Dl	=	deciliter
IU	=	international unit
G	=	gram
Ng	=	nanogram

Various labs may use units of measure that are different from the ones given in the charts. As a result, the normal ranges may need to be adjusted to that specific lab's units of measure.

Lab Values Reference Table

Lab Value	Normal Ranges	Significance	What Can An Advocate Do?
Albumin	3.3-5 g/dl	Albumin is a component of body proteins. A decrease in albumin is an indicator that nutrition may be deficient and there is a lack of protein in the diet.	Ask if foods high in protein, such as meats, cheese and beans, are in the diet. Can other supplements help elevate the protein level?
Arterial Blood Gases	PH 7.35 -7.45 PO2 80 – 100 PCO2 35-45 HCO3 2 2 – 26	This test measures how well the blood is oxygenated, and is often done when someone has respiratory problems. Patients who are on a ventilator (breathing machine) will have blood gases drawn.	Be sure the patient has his/her head elevated because breathing will be easier. Oxygen is usually not given unless the PO2 is less than 90.
Blood urea nitrogen (BUN)	5 – 25 mg/dl	Increased levels may indicate kidney problems or dehydration.	Provided there are not problems with the kidneys, increasing fluids may help decrease the levels.
Creatinine	0.5-1.5 mg/dl	This test is done to diagnose kidney dysfunction. Some drugs may increase the levels.	If impaired kidney function is suspected, ask the teams if fluids need to be limited.

Lab Value	Normal Ranges	Significance	What Can An Advocate Do?
Cultures	Negative	Cultures are taken to see if there are bacteria in body tissues or fluids. Results are helpful in prescribing antibiotics. Antibiotics are started before the results are returned.	The cultures may not come back for a few days. When the results are given, there may be a change in the choice of antibiotics.
Enzymes **CPK, HBD, LDH, SGOT, SGPT**	Individual norms are under the individually listed section.	Enzyme studies are used to detect cell damage and location as overactive. Diseased or injured cells increase the release of enzymes into the plasma.	You may hear the team talk about enzymes in general. If you are interested, ask about which values are abnormal.
Glucose or blood sugar **Fasting – nothing to eat 12 hours before Post prandial – 2 hours after a meal.**	70 - 110 mg/dl	Elevated levels may indicate diabetes, stress, use of steroids, infection or use of certain medications. Low levels may indicate starvation or too much insulin given by injection.	Blood sugars are watched very closely during hospital stays. Check with the team to be sure that food brought in will not contribute to fluctuations in the result.

Lab Value	Normal Ranges	Significance	What Can An Advocate Do?
Hemato-crit (Hct)	Male 40-54% Female 36-46%	The hematocrit measures the number of red blood cells in 100 milliliters of blood. Low levels may indicate anemia, leukemia or over-hydration. A high count may indicate dehydration, or increased numbers of red blood cells, which may result in "thick blood".	Ask if you can help with increasing or decreasing fluids as indicated by the level.
Hemo-globin (Hb or Hgb)	Male 13.5 – 17 g/dl Female 12 – 15 g/dl	Measures the amount of hemoglobin in the blood and is one of the best determinants of anemia.	Ask if a trans-fusion is needed and/or if iron has been prescribed or what foods may help increase iron levels.
INR ratio- Interna-tional Sensitivity Index	0.8 – 1.3 seconds Recom-mended therapeutic range: 2.0 – 3.5	Proposed reporting format when prothrombin time is utilized; this is used with the drug Warfarin (Coumadin). Therapeutic ranges vary, depending on degree of blood thinning desired.	INR monitoring is extremely important to determine the correct dosage of Coumadin. Coumadin therapy can be very dangerous if levels are not monitored carefully. Watch for signs of abnormal bleeding.

Lab Value	Normal Ranges	Significance	What Can An Advocate Do?
Magnesium	1.2 - 2.5 mEq/L	Magnesium controls sodium, potassium, calcium and phosphorus. It also functions in the utilization of carbohydrates, lipids and proteins, which activate enzyme systems that enable B vitamins to function. It is also essential for nucleic acid synthesis and blood clotting.	If other values such as sodium and potassium are abnormal, ask if the magnesium has been checked. The magnesium has to be corrected before the others will correct.
Partial Thrombo-Plastin Time (PTT)	60 – 70 seconds. May vary with different labs.	Measures the effects of certain blood thinners; when Heparin is being used, the ranges need to be higher than indicated if blood thinning is occurring.	Check for signs of bleeding – easy bruising, blood in the urine, or nosebleeds.
Potassium	3.5 - 5.3 mEq/L	Essential for the transmission of electrical impulses in the heart and skeletal muscle. High or low potassium may have an effect on heart rhythm. Low levels may result in nausea, irregular pulse, dizziness, leg cramps, muscle weakness, or affect heart rhythm; High levels may lead to a slow pulse, numbness of hands or legs or affect heart rhythm.	High or low Potassium levels may affect the heart. Check for changes in the rhythm (spacing of beats) of the pulse.

Lab Value	Normal Ranges	Significance	What Can An Advocate Do?
Prealbumin	17 - 40 mg/dl	The risk of protein calorie malnutrition for hospitalized patients can be as high as 50%. Prealbumin has been used as an aid in earlier assessment and intervention of nutritional problems and malnutrition.	What is being done to help nutrition? Is the patient getting enough food, and/or supplemental feedings? Can I bring food from home?
Protein	6.0-8.0 g/dl	Decreased total protein is seen in malnutrition, liver disease, burns, Crohn's disease, diabetes, and malnutrition. Low protein can cause swelling in the feet and hands.	What is being done to maintain proper nutrition? Is the patient getting enough food, and/or supplemental feedings? Can I bring food from home?
Prothrombin time (PT) or Pro-Time	10 – 13 seconds	Measures the effect of the drug Coumadin. Vitamin K reverses the effect. The INR is usually done to determine drug dosages. When on Coumadin, the lab value needs to be longer than 13 seconds to show that blood thinning is occurring. The INR is a better standard for treatment than the PT as a stand-alone test.	If the patient is on Coumadin to help thin the blood, be sure that green leafy vegetables are not given, as they reverse the effect of the drug. Look for signs of bleeding, such as on the gums, or bruising, which may necessitate a change in dosage.

Lab Value	Normal Ranges	Significance	What Can An Advocate Do?
Sodium	135 - 145 mEq/L	Sodium, or salt, plays a major role in maintaining fluid balance in the body. Increased levels may be seen in dehydration, while decreased levels may be seen with over-hydration.	Symptoms of low sodium are anxiety, muscle twitching, weakness, and headaches. Avoid drinking plain water. Symptoms of high sodium are restlessness, thirst, and dry tongue. Encourage an increase in fluids and foods low in salt.
Urine	Should look clear and yellow	Abnormal findings in the urine are sugar and bacteria.	If you see a change in urine color, blood in the urine, or clumps, ask questions. If there is a catheter (tube from the bladder), look at the color often. Be careful however, because the tubing can stain a dark color, resembling sediment.
WBC - White Blood Cell Count	4.5-10 thousand	WBCs are the primary defense of the body and increase in number if infection is present.	When high, there may be infection. Wash your hands carefully. If low, the patient may be susceptible to infection. Do not, under any circumstances come into contact with the patient if you are ill.

Common Diagnostic Tests

Prior to having a diagnostic test, it is important that you and the patient are aware of the correct preparation. Some diagnostic tests require that the bowels be cleared the day before the examination. Other tests may require that nothing be taken by mouth for up to 14 hours prior to the test.

It is important to ask the health team what preparations may be necessary. As the advocate, ask what you can do to help the patient become prepared.

Additional tests are located in Appendix G.

Test and Purpose	Procedure	Where Done	Comments/ Aftercare
Angiography - To detect aneurysms, clots and lesions in blood vessels	A catheter is placed in a vessel and a dye is flushed.	Radiology, special lab, or surgery	Patient may need to lie flat for a few hours after the procedure.
Biopsy – to identify a disease process or malignancy	Body tissue is removed surgically and examined by a pathologist.	Office or surgery	Some biopsies may take weeks to get a result.
Colonoscopy- To detect bleeding in the lower gastrointestinal tract. To look for polyps in the large intestine, and to screen for tumors in the colon.	The GI tract will need to be cleared with laxatives or enemas. Mild sedation is provided as a large tube is inserted into the rectum to directly visualize the colon.	GI lab	Patient usually lies on their left side for the procedure. The patient usually doesn't remember too much of the exam, since some sedation is given. Some mild discomfort may be experienced.

Test and Purpose	Procedure	Where Done	Comments/ Aftercare
CT or CAT Scan - to screen for coronary artery disease, (CAD), head, liver, kidney lesions, tumors, swelling, abscesses, infection, cancer, vascular problems, stroke or bone destruction. Also done to locate foreign objects in soft tissues.	CT scans the body looking at cross sections with a donut-shaped device that surrounds the body part. The exam does not hurt in any way, but may be loud. Some patients complain of claustrophobia.	Radiology	If you know the patient may be claustrophobic, let the technician know. Help the patient with relaxation techniques, as the patient needs to be very still during the exam. May or may not be done with a contrast material. If done with contrast, an I.V. will be started to inject the material. Results need to come from the physician, so don't bother asking the technician.
EKG, ECG, Electrocardiography - determines heart rhythm, electrolyte imbalances, heart rhythm changes during stress, and heart chamber enlargement	Electrodes are attached to the arms, legs and chest.	Bedside, office, or in the cardiology area	May be done on a treadmill or bicycle. Does not cause any type of electrical shock.

Test and Purpose	Procedure	Where Done	Comments/ Aftercare
EGD, Esophogastro- duodenoscopy - to examine the esophagus, stom- ach and duo- denum; obtain specimens and check for disease	A large tube with a scope at- tached is placed in the mouth. The tube is then threaded into the esophagus, stomach and the first part of the small intestine, called the duodenum. The patient is sedated and will probably not re- member most of what occurred.	G.I. lab	The patient receives medication during the procedure to help with sedation.
GI Series, Upper GI Series, Barium swallow - to detect esopha- geal, gastric or duodenal ulcers, polyps, tumors, foreign bodies, esophageal bleeds or a hiatal hernia	A large tube is placed into the mouth, and then the esophagus and duodenum.	GI Lab	The patient is awake, but sedated.
IVP – intravenous pyelography - looks at the size, shape and functioning of the kidneys in order to detect stones, tumors, or cysts.	An I.V. will need to be started. A dye is flushed in the I.V., which then is visual- ized by x-ray.	Radiology	May feel flushing and a salty or metallic taste during the injection.

Test and Purpose	Procedure	Where Done	Comments/ Aftercare
MRI – Magnetic Resonance Imaging - detects problems with the blood vessels, blood flow, central nervous system, injury, tumors or swelling.	Like the CT, the MRI looks at cross sections of the body. The device may be noisy. If the patient is claustrophobic, be sure to let the technician know.	Radiology	Alert the team if the patient has any metal devices in the body, as the magnet may pull on these. The machine makes a lot of clicking noises; the patient may feel a tingling in dental fillings.
X-Ray - examines bone structure and tissue in the body.	Non-invasive procedure using a picture-taking machine.	Radiology	The patient may need to wait a few minutes after the test to make sure the films are readable.

Bedside Story

In reviewing Hilda's medical record after she became so ill, I noted that she had a very low sodium level when she was discharged from the hospital and transferred to the rehabilitation facility. When Hilda arrived at the rehabilitation facility, she was extremely ill for about one week. Intensive medical treatment was required to stabilize her condition.

If I had known at the time that her sodium level was so low, I would have questioned the transfer and insisted that it be delayed. Unfortunately, at that time, we were so excited and eager to begin rehabilitation, we did not think to ask what her lab values were.

When someone is being transferred to a level of care that generally takes less nursing oversight, ask if the lab values and diagnostic tests are stable enough for transfer. Some lab values can be slightly abnormal without causing big problems, while others are critical. As an advocate, one is not expected to know this, but the general question of "How do the lab values seem? How are the vital signs?" may provide an additional assessment to double check that transfer is appropriate.

*Key Points

- Carry a resource with you on basic lab values.

- Ask the medical team if the lab values are within normal limits. This may remind the medical team to review the values.

- Most important values to know are the WBC, Hgb, Potassium and Sodium.

- Ask questions if you do not know the significance of an abnormal value.

- Always question the reason for a diagnostic test to be sure the test is intended for your loved one.

Notes

_____

_____

_____

_____

_____

_____

_____

_____

_____

_____

_____

_____

_____

_____

_____

_____

_____

_____

Nutrition First

The doctors focus on the tests,
And medicine and drugs and rest.
Nutrition though, and food will be
Essential for recovery.

If you don't like the food that's served,
And what's at home might have more verve;
Just ask the family and all friends,
Your favorites bring to help you mend.

Load up on proteins, fiber too;
And fats as well, you should accrue.
It's too important to ignore
Please "eat to heal" we do implore.

CHAPTER 7
Nutrition First

Nutritional care and support is one area of intervention in which you <u>must</u> actively participate. Do not delay in asking about the nutritional status of the patient and what you can do to help. When a patient is seriously ill, priority is given to medications and diagnostic tests. By the time the patient's nutritional needs are addressed, irreversible damage might have already occurred.

Malnutrition in the hospitalized patient can occur primarily as a result of reduced or no food intake. The seriousness of this deprivation is compounded by the increased energy expenditure as the body fights the disease or illness. As the patient's metabolism increases, the body needs more proteins for healing and the functioning of organs. Thus, hospitalized patients will suffer specifically from calorie and protein malnutrition.

Malnutrition impacts all aspects of a patient's care and recovery. Among them are the following:

- Increased chances for infection as malnutrition lowers the body's resistance to disease
- Delays the healing process
- Leads to skin breakdown
- Increases the severity and complicates the management of chronic conditions
- Reduces the patient's physical abilities
- Impairs mental functioning
- Results in eventual deterioration and death

Poor nutrition is a common, potentially serious and under-recognized problem among all patients, but affects hospitalized older patients more adversely. According to an article in the June 2, 1999 issue of the *Journal of the American Medical Association (JAMA)*, Dennis H. Sullivan M.D., of the Central Arkansas Veterans Healthcare System in Little Rock, Arkansas and his colleagues studied 497 patients, 65-years old or older, who were hospitalized for four days or more. Their findings were extremely disturbing:

- (21%) of these elderly patients consumed less than 50% of their calculated maintenance energy requirements.

- The low-nutrient group was eight times as likely to die in the hospital, and almost three times as likely to die within 90 days of discharge.

- Many of these patients had orders for (NPO) nothing by mouth throughout much of their hospitalization without being given alternative forms of nutritional support.

- In short, although the researchers did not state it so succinctly, the patients were virtually starved to death.

- According to the report, up to 60% of elderly hospitalized patients are protein-energy undernourished on admission or develop serious nutritional deficits prior to discharge.

All patients, regardless of age, however, are possible candidates for having malnutrition, as there are factors present in every hospital that will contribute to the development of this condition.

The first factor is the procedure used by most hospitals when the patient first arrives. Patients who are critically ill or severely injured are usually given only I.V. fluids upon admission. This occurs so that doctors provide treatment and administer various tests for diagnostic purposes. One liter of I.V. fluid of 5% dextrose and water contains only 200 calories. A patient may receive about 2 liters of this mixture per day, yielding the patient a total daily caloric intake of 400 calories. If the testing covers a two-day span, the patient will have had a total of 800 calories. Also, keep in mind that the person who is hospitalized often has not eaten the day he or she was admitted. This results in the patient receiving 800 calories over three days when he or she would normally have probably eaten a minimum of 5000 in that same time span. Ironically, at the very time when patients need more calories to promote healing, they are receiving less.

Other factors also play an important role in preventing patients from becoming malnourished. Chief among these is the failure of members of the medical plan to recognize that attention must be paid to the patient's nutritional needs. Patients commonly do not eat in a hospital for any number of reasons. Mental and organic stress, changed feeding patterns, strange foods, unfamiliar people and a hospital environment all lead to a lack of desire to eat. The medical staff needs to provide various feeding options and a selection of foods that will encourage the patient to eat and subsequently heal more quickly.

In addition, various members of the medical staff can introduce procedures that decrease the possibility that malnutrition will occur. These include the following:

• Weighing the patient daily to check types of foods and fluids

• Developing a nutritional plan for the patient

• Providing additional nutrients if the patient has been on a prolonged administration of dextrose and electrolyte-containing solutions

• Ensuring that the patient does not become dehydrated

Patients must have key elements if malnutrition is to be avoided: (1) water - dehydration may occur from the decreased intake of fluids; (2) proteins - many body tissues are composed of proteins; therefore, the protein requirement is increased for many sick patients as their bodies recover from illness or injury; (3) vitamins and minerals - to replace those that might have been lost; (4) calories - additional energy that supports the healing process.

These needs are essential regardless of the type of feeding the patient is receiving. If the patient is on intravenous feeding because either the patient cannot eat or the gastrointestinal system cannot be used, then total parenteral nutrition (TPN), where all nutrition is provided via the intravenous should be instituted as soon as possible. The same would be true if the patient is undergoing enteral feeding where the patient is fed through a tube in the nose or abdomen.

There are certain lab tests that can be used to check a patient's nutritional status. If caloric intake has been decreased for a period of time, malnutrition may be occurring and measures must be taken to assess the situation. The following chart provides information about the most critical tests that can be ordered if malnutrition is suspected.

Lab Studies to Assess Nutrition

Lab Test	Comments	Normal Ranges
Albumin	This is a protein that lives in the body for a long time. When the albumin is low, there has been malnutrition for a long period of time, and as a result, is not a reliable indicator for early malnutrition.	Greater than 3.5 g/dL
Blood urea nitrogen (BUN)	Increased levels indicate dehydration and subsequent kidney problems.	5 – 25 mg/dl
C – reactive protein (CRP)	The CRP may help to monitor the stress response which may indicate the need for further nutritional assessment.	Usually below 1 mg/dL
Creatinine	This test is also done to diagnose kidney problems or dehydration. Certain drugs may increase the levels. If creatinine levels are high, kidney functions may be impaired.	0.5 – 1.5 mg/dl
Glucose or blood sugar	Low levels of glucose may be an indication of malnutrition.	70 – 110 mg/dl

Lab Test	Comments	Normal Ranges
Magnesium	Magnesium controls sodium, potassium, calcium, and phosphorus and functions in the utilization of carbohydrates and proteins.	1.2 – 2.5 mEq/L
Prealbumin	This protein lives for a short time in the body and is a very sensitive indicator of protein deficiency.	20 – 40 mg/dL
Protein	Decreased total protein is seen in malnutrition.	6.0 – 8.0 g/dl
Retinol-binding protein (RPB)	This test is helpful in diagnosing protein malnutrition.	3 – 6 mg/dL
Sodium	Increased levels may indicate that the patient is dehydrated.	135 – 145 mEq/L
Transferrin	The transferrin reflects nutritional support better than albumin. The levels help measure iron stores. Testing the transferrin helps with the correlation of iron values.	225 – 400 mf/dl

If the lab values are outside of the normal ranges, you should take several actions: (1) ask for a dietary consult; (2) ask for supplemental drinks that are high in protein; (3) ask if you can bring in protein bars; (4) after a few days, ask the physician if the lab values can be rechecked.

Using lab values is only one means for checking for signs of malnutrition. Observation is another. Patients who might be suffering from malnutrition could exhibit some or any of the following signs, depending upon whether the patient is at high or moderate risk.

Symptom	Signs of Moderate Risk	Signs of High Risk	What You Can Do
Decreased Physical and Mental Functioning	Needs help to get out of bed. Tremors Needs some assistance with eating, chewing or swallowing Teeth in poor repair Dentures that don't fit well. Limited ability to communicate.	Bedridden Total dependence upon others for eating Tube feedings Mouth pain	Be present to help with eating meals. If there are problems with the teeth, ask for soft or puréed foods. Ask if you can bring food from home.
Skin Condition	Redness, blisters or a break in the skin. Inability to control urine or bowel movement.	A bedsore that is down to the muscle or bone. Multiple bed sores.	As soon as there is ANY redness or break in the skin, contact the nurse and ask that skin care protection procedures be initiated. Do not massage directly over red areas of the skin. This may cause more damage. After urinating or bowel movement, make sure that the skin is properly cleansed. Special mattress, turning every 2 hours, and range of motion are ESSENTIAL in prevention of breakdown. Nutrition and hydration are also very helpful.

Symptom	Signs of Moderate Risk	Signs of High Risk	What You Can Do
Weight Status	A 5% change in weight over 30 days.	Greater than 5% weight change in 30 days.	Request that daily weights be taken. Double check to be sure that the weights are done at the same time of the day with the same amount of clothes. If there is continued weight loss, ask to speak to the dietician to see how caloric intake can be increased.
Food Intake	Less than 75%	Less than 25%	Find out what food he/she likes. Help with eating. Ask to bring foods from home. Offer foods in small portions throughout the day. Give praise for eating. If foods are hard to eat, ask for protein shakes.
Fluid Intake	Less than 1 1/2 quarts per day.	Less than 1 quart per day.	Ask the nursing staff to monitor and record the intake and output of fluids. Check the patient's mouth. If it is dry, this is a sign that dehydration is occurring.
Medication Intake	Taking more than two to four drugs per day.	Taking more than five different drugs per day.	Many medications may affect appetite. Try to offer nutritious foods in small portions during the day. Ask if high protein or caloric shakes can be provided.

Symptom	Signs of Moderate Risk	Signs of High Risk	What You Can Do
Diagnoses	High Blood Pressure, Diabetes, Low Blood Counts, Stroke, Urinary Tract Infection, Alcohol or drug abuse, recent surgery, food intolerances, constipation, diarrhea, Reflux Disease, Parkinson's.	Cancer that is advanced, liver failure, dialysis, Alzheimer's, dementia, depression, dehydration, difficulty swallowing, bleeding from the stomach or bowels, nausea, vomiting.	If one of these diseases is present, you must be alert very early on to nutritional deficiencies. Ask the physician if protein levels have been checked. If you suspect nutritional concerns early, request that prealbumin levels be checked. Request a dietary consult if there is concern.

As an advocate for the patient, your observations and actions will be one of the most important tools in helping a patient avoid the onset of malnutrition. In the following chart, there are some problems patients often exhibit and suggested ways for you to become involved in helping to alleviate or ameliorate that problem or condition.

Problem	What You Can Do
Chewing Problems	• Ask for soft, ground, puréed or liquid food. • Offer small bites. • Have the person sit up to eat. • Follow food with fluid.
Constipation	• Encourage fluids. • Emphasize foods high in fiber. • Encourage fruits, vegetables, whole-grain breads and cereals. • Increase activity. • Ask if there are medications, such as narcotics, that may be causing the constipation. • Ask if there are any laxatives or stool softeners ordered.

Problem	What You Can Do
Decreased appetite	• Eat at regular meals. • Use foods high in calories. • Help make the environment comfortable. • Ask about bringing foods from home.
Decreased sensation of smell or taste	• Ask if seasonings may be added. • Provide colorful and attractive foods. • Avoid use of inhaler medications before mealtimes. • Decrease or avoid smoking.
Diarrhea	• Ask if there may be lactose intolerance. • Consider that there may be a medical cause for the diarrhea. • Ask about common medications, such as antibiotics, antacids, tranquilizers, diuretics and antidepressant meds, which may cause this side effect. • Limit use of caffeine. • Make sure there is adequate fluid intake. • Bananas and yogurt may help with some forms of diarrhea.
Dry Mouth	• Use tart liquids, such as lemonade or cranberry juice. • Use sugarless candy to stimulate saliva. • Add soup, gravy or milk to food to increase moisture. • Medicated lip balm can be very helpful to soothe dry lips. However, if oxygen is being administered, do not use a product containing petroleum.
Iron Deficiency	• Avoid fluids, such as tea and coffee, with meal. • Eat iron-rich foods.
Swallowing problems	• Check for swallowing problems, such as pocketing of food in cheeks, coughing during or after foods, liquid or medications. • Modify food consistency to aid with swallowing. Foods that are a pudding consistency are easier to swallow. • Sit up for eating. • May request a referral with a speech therapist to assess swallowing ability.

Some patients face the additional problem of having restricted diets that limit or prohibit eating certain foods. The following charts provide information on what foods to avoid, depending upon the type of diet a patient has been assigned.

These charts are particularly important if family and friends have been given permission and encouragement to bring food from home.

Restriction	Foods to Avoid
Fat Restricted	• Milk, cream, ice cream • Biscuits, pancakes, cakes, granola, chips, stuffing, fried tortillas, cornbread • Cakes, cookies, pies, pastries, puddings, cream puffs • Avocados • Canned fish packed in oil, duck, breaded poultry, cutlets, ribs, corned beef, ground beef, hot dogs, and luncheon meats, such as bologna, and salami • More than 1 egg yolk per day • Cheeses, such as American, blue, brie, cheddar, Jack or Swiss • Fried potatoes, fried rice, chow mein noodles • Buttered or creamed vegetables
Fiber Restricted	• Yogurt with seeds or nuts • Any whole-grain bread, graham crackers, cornbread • Oatmeal, bran, anything with seeds or nuts • Dried fruit, all berries, raw fruits with membranes, prune juice • Corn, vegetables with seeds • Nuts, coconut, popcorn, pickles
Sodium (salt) restricted diet	• Vegetable or tomato juices • Crackers and breads with salted tops • Salad dressings with bacon bits • Any smoked, cured, salted, koshered or canned meat, fish, or poultry • Commercially-prepared potatoes, rice or pasta mixes • Canned soups • Vegetables prepared in brine • Any seasoning made with salt, soy sauce, and teriyaki sauce

If the medical team has given permission and encouragement for family members and friends to bring food from home, the chart below provides suggestions, depending upon what type of diet the patient is following.

Diet	Foods to Encourage
Calcium Rich diet	• Yogurt, milk, cheese and tofu • Calcium-fortified orange juice • Cheese pizza • Cheddar cheese • Canned salmon with edible bones • Macaroni and cheese
High Calorie - High Protein	• All hot cereals with milk, granola • All vegetables with added fat • Canned fruits in heavy syrup, dried fruit • All fried meats, meats in sauces • Whole milk, ice cream, cheese, whipping cream • All creamed and meat soups • All oils, butter, margarine, mayonnaise, bacon, avocado, salad dressings, cream cheese, sour cream
High-calorie suggestions	• Melt butter or margarine on potatoes, hot cereals, rice, noodles and vegetables • Add sour cream to any cooked potatoes, pastas or casseroles • Mayonnaise on sandwiches or crackers • Spread cream cheese on fruit slices, raw vegetables, bread or luncheon meats • Use half and half cream instead of milk or water in soups, sauces, custards and puddings • Serve heavy whipping cream on fruit, ice cream, pudding or Jell-O • Add brown sugar, maple syrup or honey to cereals, puddings or vegetables
High Fiber	• Apples, bran, peanuts, pears, peas, bananas, corn • Cabbage, cauliflower, grapes • Dried beans, green beans, oak bran, oatmeal, and sesame seeds

Diet	Foods to Encourage
High-Protein Intake	• Melt cheese on hamburgers, hot dogs and other meats • Add cheese to sandwiches, sauces and casseroles • Spread peanut butter on toast, sandwiches, and crackers; blend into milkshakes, yogurt or ice cream • Use eggs as much as possible • Add ice cream to milkshakes or sodas • Add meats to soups, omelets, casseroles, and sandwiches • Add nuts to ice cream, puddings, muffins or cookies • Look for yogurt made from whole milk • Add beans, peas and lentils to soups, casseroles and dips • All kinds of tofu are very good
Increased Potassium Diet	• Peas, beans, lentils • Bran, gingerbread, granola • Cheese • Apricots, bananas, cantaloupe, dates, figs, mango, orange juice • Artichokes, avocado, potatoes • Pumpkin, spinach • Salt substitutes, chili sauce, barbecue sauce
Iron-Rich Diet	• Clams, oysters, liver, chicken, beef, dark meat, turkey • Canned lima, red kidney beans and split peas • Cooked enriched egg noodles • Dried apricots • Cooked beans, breakfast cereals enriched with iron

Drugs may also play a role in a patient's developing malnutrition, as they often affect appetite, sense of smell and taste. Some drugs will interact negatively with various foods and liquids. The following chart lists some common types of drugs and any food or liquid restrictions that accompany the use of each.

Drug Types	Examples	Comments
Antibacterials, Gastric Acid Reducers	• Penicillin and derivatives • Zithromax • Didanosine • Indinavir • Fosamax • Prevacid	Should be taken at least 1 hour prior to a meal on an empty stomach.
Calcium channel blockers	• Plendil, Adalat, Procardia, Nimotop, Calan, Isoptin	Avoid taking grapefruit juice, as it increases the drug levels.
Coumadin	• Warfarin	Limit foods high in vitamin K to one serving per day. This includes beef liver, green leafy vegetables, brussels sprouts, broccoli or soybean oil.
Diuretics	• Drugs that increase fluid from the body, such as Lasix (Furosemide) and Bumex (Bumetanide)	Eat foods high in potassium, such as apricots, broccoli, dates, sweet potatoes, oranges, tomatoes, prunes, raisins, milk, potatoes, bananas, mushrooms, melons, avocados and asparagus.
Lithium Products	• Eskalith, Lithobid, Lithionate, Lithium Carbonate	Maintain a diet that includes a consistent salt intake and drink at least 8 to 10 glasses of water each day.
MAO Inhibitors	• Drugs such as Nardil, Parnate, or Marplan	Avoid the following: • aged cheeses or cheese products • dried, salted, pickled, smoked or fermented meats • yeast extracts • fava bread or Italian beans • red wines, beer, ale, vermouth, sherry • sourdough and fresh homemade yeast-leavened breads

Drug Types	Examples	Comments
Pain Relief	• Percocet • Percodan • Ferrous sulfate • Tylenol with codeine • Morphine • Vicodin	May cause constipation
Tetracyclines	• Achromycin, Vibramycin, Cipro, Floxin, Levaquin, Niazoral	Avoid antacids (such as Maalox, Mylanta, Tums), iron and dairy products within one hour of taking these medications.

Bedside Story

Hilda, nutritionally, was in great shape prior to her hospitalization. Believe me, no one in our family has wanted for lack of nutrition! Yet, within one week after her surgery, she began to develop bed sores, which are a type of skin breakdown and a common result of malnutrition. Hilda had lain on her back for quite awhile after surgery, yet even our conscientious turning could not prevent the horrendous bed sore that refused to heal. Of course, I did not know that she had retained dressings in her surgical wound that made healing impossible.

What I did not know was that Hilda's sodium and protein levels had decreased drastically. Protein is very important in keeping skin intact and a simple lab test of her albumin levels could determine malnutrition within as few as three days. If I had checked those lab values, I might have been able to detect the beginnings of malnutrition.

We tried everything to reverse the process. We fed Hilda protein bars until she was sick of them. We gave her nutritional supplements of every shape and form. We pleaded and prodded, begged and cajoled. Yet, once her nutritional status began to decline, it was impossible to reverse the process.

*Key Points

- Nutrition is a priority. You need to advocate early to ensure your patient is getting the proper nutrition.

- If your patient does not like hospital food, get permission from the staff to bring favorite foods from home.

- If food is brought from home, observe all diet restrictions.

- If you believe nutritional needs are not being addressed, ask for a dietary consultation. The dieticians are wonderful in assessing and making recommendations.

- Help the patient with eating. Be there for meal times if you can. Help make the room pleasant by making sure the environment is clean and odor-free.

- Praise the patient for increased food consumption.

- When the skin begins to break down, alert staff immediately. Take pictures of the breakdown so that you can document its progress.

- Ask to see lab values on protein and pre-albumin levels.

- Turning the patient frequently can help prevent skin deterioration.

- If available, special mattresses can help prevent the development of bed sores.

Notes

_____

_____

_____

_____

_____

_____

_____

_____

Notes

"Who Cares?"
Care you can Give
in the Hospital

The simple tasks that life demands,
For some require helping hands.
An incapacitated friend
Needs lots of care that you can tend.

It can be quite a tricky feat
To turn someone or change a sheet.
Or bathe a person lying down
Before you change their sleeping gown.

To keep the muscles from decay,
There's exercises done each day.
These "range of motion" moves are tough,
But help to keep the body "buff".

CHAPTER 8
"Who Cares?" Care You Can Give in the Hospital

There are many things that you can do to help care for your loved one. Helping with basic care allows you to feel productive, gives you time with your loved one, and can be a big help to the medical team. Described below are the various procedures that can be done and how to perform each task. Be sure to check with the medical team first and have them assist you with getting prepared.

Hand washing – A Must-Do Activity!

The hospital environment is loaded with new bacteria to which you and your loved one have never been exposed. Some of these bacteria are resistant to treatment by antibiotics; therefore, the infections they cause can be very serious. Hand washing is the single most significant protection in the spread of bacteria.

Procedure:

- Remove jewelry and push your watch to the mid-forearm or remove it.
- Turn on the water to a warm temperature.
- Run hands under water, keeping your hands in a downward position.
- Apply liquid soap and lather.
- Rub hands together for 10-15 seconds and wash between fingers and under nails.
- Rinse hands with the hands in a downward position.
- Dry hands in the direction of fingers to wrists.
- Turn faucet off with a clean, dry paper towel.

Changing Sheets with Your Loved One in the Bed

If you want to help put clean sheets on the bed, be sure you check with the medical team. Initially, helping the nurse will give you a good idea of the procedure. If you think you may be taking care of your loved one at home, the hospital is a great place to start practicing.

Procedure:

Depending upon how soiled the sheets are, you may want to wear gloves during this procedure.

- Make sure the bed rail is up on the far side of the bed.

- Remove the top sheet.

- Ask the patient to turn on their side, away from you.

- Untuck the soiled sheet and roll it toward the middle of the bed into the form of a sausage.

- The clean sheet is then placed on the empty side of the bed. The sheet is tucked in the side nearest to you with the untucked portion rolled into the form of a second sausage lying in the middle of the bed.

- Once you have the two rolls of sheets, side by side, ask the patient to roll back toward you over both rolls of linen.

- Put up the bed rail on the side of the bed where you have been standing, and go around to the other side of the bed.

- Take down the bed rail. Pull the soiled sheet off the bed; then pull the clean sheet through, smooth it out and tuck it in.

- Place soiled linen in a hamper.

- Be sure to wash your hands when you are finished if you have not worn gloves.

Bathing your Loved One in Bed

The first rule of bathing a patient in bed is that he or she should do as much for himself or herself as possible. If you are to help, be sure you talk with the nurse first to find out what you should do. Bathing in the hospital may take various forms because, while hygiene is extremely important, not everyone needs a full bath each day. A partial bath, which includes face, armpits and groin may be all that is necessary. Hair is washed only if there is a physician's order to do so. If the patient is allowed to take a shower, the nurse will help with this activity. The procedure described below is implemented when the patient is to receive a complete bed bath.

Procedure:

- Make sure you have washed your hands.

- Provide for privacy by pulling curtains and/or closing doors.

- If needed, use gloves.

- If a bath blanket (a soft, lightweight blanket) is available, place the bath blanket over your loved one and wash areas as you come to them. If a bath blanket is not available, use the top sheet to cover the person.

- Fill the washbasin 2/3 full and check the temperature. Ask your loved one how the temperature feels. You will be changing the water whenever a soap film develops, or the water becomes contaminated.

- It is helpful to have at least 2 washcloths, one for soap and one for rinsing, and at least one towel.

- Each body part should be washed, rinsed, and dried in the order listed on the chart.

Body Part	Procedure
Face, neck and ears	Wipe eyes from inside to outside using a clean part of the washcloth.
Arms, forearms and hands	Use long strokes towards the body, and then wash the armpit. The arm may need to be supported while you wash.
Chest and abdomen	Use long, firm strokes. For females, clean under each breast by lifting gently.
Legs and feet	Bend the leg at the knee, starting with the leg farthest from you. Wash with long strokes towards the body. Do not ever massage the legs. If desired, you may soak the feet in the wash basin. Consider changing the water.
Back	Have your loved one lie on their side, or if allowed, on the stomach. Use long strokes from the buttocks towards the head. Use lotion for a backrub.
Groin area	Use a clean washcloth. It is best if the person can do this for themselves, but if not, you may assist if you have your loved one's permission. • Male – wash gently around the penis and scrotum, making sure areas are dried. Wash the anal area last. • Female – wash from front to back, making sure areas are dried. Wash the anal area last.

Apply deodorant as needed.

Help dress the patient in a clean gown.

The bed sheets should be changed after the bath.

Turning
- Turning helps prevent bed sores, increases circulation, and may help prevent pneumonia.
- All patients must be turned at least every 2 hours.
- Ask the staff to demonstrate proper techniques for turning the patient.
- With any lifting or turning, bend your knees so you will not hurt your back.

Exercises that Can be Done in Bed

After getting permission from the medical team, ask what can be done to help with physical activity. Muscles can actually shorten overnight from lack of activity and can stiffen or weaken to a point where normal function cannot be returned. Exercise can help send needed oxygen to tissues and improve circulation. Exercise also helps prevent blood clots.

Range of motion is a technique that requires patients to move most of their muscle groups. Make sure that you always get permission to do range of motion with the patient to be sure that you are not stressing body parts that shouldn't be moved. Range of motion should be done several times a day and is best done if the patient can move the muscle groups themselves, but there are times when you may need to assist, because the patient cannot move them on their own. To learn how to do range of motion on the patient, practice the following moves for yourself first so that you know the moves! Perform each technique at least three times.

- Move your head to your chin and then back. Turn your head in a circle.

- Take your arms and straighten them out and then flex a few times.

- Stretch your fingers out and then bend them back and forth.

- Move your arms in a circle.

- Move your wrists in a circle.

- Bend your knees and then straighten out your legs.

- Move your hips in a circle.

- Move your foot back and forwards and in a circle.

If the patient can't move their feet, it is very important that the feet are placed in a position so that there is a bend at the ankle. When a patient cannot move his or her feet, the ligament can actually stretch and cause a condition caused "foot drop". To prevent this from occurring, place a pillow against the end of the feet to keep them bent at the ankles. When a person is paralyzed, you can ask for permission to bring in high top tennis shoes that can be worn in bed. This intervention keeps the feet bent and can prevent foot drop.

If you find that your loved one is not moving around enough, or that muscles seem to be stiffening, ask for a physical therapy consultation. The physical therapist will be able to develop an appropriate exercise program for the patient.

Bedside Story

Hilda needed help with most of her basic care. This was an area where I really felt that I could help, as I really enjoyed assisting with her bathing and performing range of motion exercises. Range of motion was a must for Hilda. Since she was paralyzed from her chest down, she was unable to move her legs or lower body. I started range of motion with her right away. I didn't want her legs to look deformed as we envisioned that day when she would be wheeling herself around the beach! The staff appreciated the help. I also taught my sisters how to help with the bathing and turning. This was our way of really giving back to our mother some of the love she had given to us her whole life.

*Key Points

- Wash your hands before and after working with the patient.
- Wear gloves anytime you may be touching body fluids.
- Ask the nursing staff to show you how to do procedures before attempting the procedures on your own.
- Let the staff know that you need to know how to do these procedures to help when your loved one goes home.
- Turning the patient every 2 hours is the standard.
- Range of motion exercises are very important to help prevent stiffening of muscles. A footboard may help prevent foot drop (stretching of the ligaments of the foot).

Leaving the Hospital

Eventually, there comes the day,
The patient will be sent away.
To home or other place- to wait
Or rest or rehabilitate.

The move requires lots of thought,
As special services are sought.
The preparations must be set,
And food and nursing care to get.

If hospice care is what you face
Then comfort is to be embraced.
And efforts should be focused on
Providing love 'til life is gone.

CHAPTER 9
Leaving the Hospital

The day will come when the hospital staff decides that it is time to transfer or discharge your loved one. That decision will be based upon several factors. The primary one is the condition of the patient and the projected type of care he or she will need in order to recover. Also affecting the decision are insurance limitations or restrictions, projected length of recovery, resources that would be necessary if the patient went home, and his or her Diagnostic Related Grouping (DRG). DRG is the projected number of days that Medicare will pay for hospitalization for a certain type of injury or illness. If the patient stays beyond the DRG, the extra days are not paid for by Medicare. A hospital will always try to release a patient when his or her DRG is through.

There is a major difference between transfer and discharge. When the patient is "transferred," the hospital communicates with the receiving facility to arrange for transportation and on-going care. Depending upon the type of facility, different levels of care are provided, but regardless of facility, the care is provided by on-duty staff at the facility. Prior to the patient being discharged, it is important to look at many options and resources. The Case Manager or Social Worker can also be a helpful resource for you and your loved one.

When the patient is "discharged," family members of the patient become responsible for both care and coordinating services. It is very difficult for a single individual to handle the preparation and process required for a discharge. You need to have a team of helpers ready when the patient goes home. Moreover, if the patient is to be discharged to home, the decision should be made early enough so the caregivers can learn how to perform necessary tasks and skills safely.

The following chart outlines the various transfer and discharge options that are available:

Leaving Options	Type	Description and Considerations
Assisted Living	Discharge	Assisted living environments provide the patient with their own room or apartment where the patient can have their own belongings. Meal preparation and medication support can be provided. This can be a good option that may be less costly than 1:1 in-home care.
Home alone with family support	Discharge	Discuss the needs for your loved one. Do you have the skills to provide the necessary care? Determine if 24-hour care is needed.
Home care with private agency support, such as nurses, sitters, personal care workers, healthcare aides	Discharge	This option may work if the financial resources are available. Often, this is a good choice, as your loved one can be in a familiar environment where the necessary care can be given by experts.
Home with support from community agencies, such as Meals on Wheels, and seniors support services	Discharge	This is a mix of family support and outside agencies. These agencies only drop in for services.
Palliative Care or hospice services in the home setting.	Discharge	The patient has been determined to be terminal. Support services are similar to home care, but the emphasis is comfort and care, rather than cure for the patient.

Leaving Options	Type	Description and Considerations
Retirement Homes	Discharge	Retirement homes are privately owned and operated residences. Each home provides accommodation, meals and recreational activities. The assistance they offer varies and can include help with bathing, supervision of medication, and assistance with dressing. Assisted Living units are available in some residences at a greater cost. Some other residences do not provide a separate Assisted Living unit, but bring nursing care to your room.
Complex Continuing Care facility (chronic care) or Long-Term Acute Care	Transfer	These facilities provide intense nursing care for a long period of time. When the patient can no longer be in the acute care hospital, often due to financial limitations, transfer to this type of facility provides the necessary nursing care and services that may be covered by other types of insurance categories.
Convalescent Care for long-term or Nursing Home	Transfer	This option is chosen when the needs of the patient exceed what can be done at home. This choice may also be made for safety reasons if the patient's behavior is violent or there may be a danger to the patient at home.

Leaving Options	Type	Description and Considerations
Convalescent Care for short-term	Transfer	This type of facility can be a good interim level of care to provide necessary medication, treatments and support before going home. If this option is used it is very important to inform the patient that this is only temporary. Often, short-term stay patients are mixed in with patients who are permanent residents.
Palliative Care or hospice services in a hospital-type setting	Transfer	This type of care is provided to a patient who is terminal. There are support services for the patient and the family. The goal is to provide comfort, not cure for the patient.
Rehabilitation services, such as Geriatric, Stroke and Head Injury	Transfer	This type of facility specializes in the care needed for the patient. Similar services as those given in the hospital are provided, with intense rehabilitation and physical therapy services.
Supervised group or boarding home	Transfer	These programs offer assisted services. There are usually 6 persons living in a home that is managed by a caregiver, who helps with meals and medications. This can be a good option for 24 hour care that is less costly than 1:1 in-home care.

If your choice is to have the patient discharged to home, then the rest of this chapter is devoted to your needs.

The most important aspect of discharge is planning ahead. First, only with extensive planning can the caregivers provide a continuity of care that is so important to preventing the patient's condition from deteriorating. Moreover, extensive planning will alleviate the anxiety and fear that both patient and caregivers will feel as the patient leaves the safety net of resources that the hospital has provided. What have we forgotten? Can we really provide the necessary care? What should we expect?

Can we get the support services we need?

The caregivers must be able to answer these questions. To do so requires developing a discharge plan that includes the following actions:

(1) Involve everyone in the discharge process. The patient, caregivers, family, and medical team should all be equal partners, and all discussions should involve as many of these people as possible.

(2) Create a list of equipment and items the patient will need. If the patient cannot walk, then additional equipment will be necessary:

<u>Items to think about having available at home:</u>
- Straws that are flexible
- A baby monitor or a bell that rings easily
- A small portable T.V. that can easily fit on the bedside table
- Supplemental feedings such as Ensure
- At least 2 sets of sheets that are pretty
- A portable storage unit (3-drawer) with wheels to keep supplies
- A caregiver's schedule
- Plenty of food

<u>Items to have if the patient is paralyzed</u>:
- Electric bed that raises the head up and down
- Bedside table that has wheels than can roll under the bed
- Wheelchair with a head support that reclines
- Hydraulic lift to transfer the patient from bed to chair (these are wonderful back savers)
- Portable oxygen
- A bath or shower chair

(3) Plan how their everyday care is to be provided. Be sure that family members know what their roles are to be.

(4) Develop a list of agencies and service providers in your community. Contact them to gather details about hours, costs, and what services they provide. Begin to arrange when these services should start if you need them.

(5) Become knowledgeable about the patient's diagnosis, prognosis, medications, and treatments. Begin to practice those skills to keep the patient safe and comfortable.

(6) Develop a checklist that needs to be completed at least two days before the patient is scheduled to be discharged. The following sample was used for Hilda. A blank template can be found in Appendix H.

Task	Completed	Questions
Has discharge been discussed with the family members who need to know?	Yes	
Has written and verbal advice been given to the patient?	No	What meds and services will she need?
Have arrangements been confirmed?	Yes	
Does the caregiver understand how to use special equipment?	No	Will equipment company inservice?
Have transfer arrangements been made?	Yes	Hospital will call ambulance.
Has there been training on the hospital equipment?	No	Will company provide?
Have friends or family brought clothes at discharge?	No	Does she need additional clothing if the ambulance is transferring?

As the day of discharge approaches, additional questions will appear. For Hilda, the caregivers thought of these at the last minute and scurried around, making telephone calls and arrangements.

- How will the ambulance drivers get her upstairs?

- Will the home care person do her shopping?

- Since she is paralyzed, how will she call us for help?

- Who do we contact if she gets worse?

- Will the hospital bed fit in her bedroom or should we put the bed in the living room?

With such extensive pre-planning, the discharge day will be filled with anticipation and excitement. The patient will be eager to leave the hospital for a familiar environment full of friends and family. However, the actual process of being discharged from the hospital requires time. The physician must complete a final check with the patient to confirm that the patient is medically stable enough for discharge. Prescriptions need to be written for drugs and medical equipment. Finally, financial matters need to be resolved.

As the advocate, there is a lot you can do to help speed up this process and prevent the patient from becoming anxious and frustrated.

- Ask the nursing staff when the anticipated time of discharge may occur.

- Clarify financial matters before arriving to the unit.

- Clarify benefits and resources before going home.

- Ask for the prescriptions and have them filled BEFORE leaving the hospital, if possible.

- Ask the nursing staff to administer the last scheduled medications before leaving the hospital. This will help prevent a gap in the continuity of medications.

- Have the equipment company deliver needed items before the patient gets home. Have someone else arrange this at the home.

- Be sure that the transportation home for the patient is ready.

- Find out the following: (1) date and time of the next appointment the patient has with the doctor; (2) the time the next medications are to be given; (3) how to get help in a crisis; (4) what variables would necessitate a return to the hospital; (5) what variables would require a 911 call.

Again, with Hilda, we created a checklist to be completed on the day of discharge. A blank template is available in the Appendix.

Task	Completed	Questions
Has access to home been arranged?	Yes	
Have medication instructions been given to the patient and the caregiver?	No	Can pharmacy give info?
Have prescriptions been obtained?	Yes	
Did someone pick up the prescriptions?	Yes	
Did the nursing staff provide medications before going home?	No	Can the last dose be given?
Have community agencies been contacted?	Hospice arranged	
Is the necessary equipment in place in the home?	Yes – they delivered yesterday	Will they in-service the family?
Has a follow-up physician appointment been made?	No	Who do we call for problems?
Is transportation confirmed?	Yes	
Has the patient been given a list of when to call the physician?	No	
Has the patient or caregivers been given a list of what situations would need a 911 call?	No	If Hilda is on hospice, do we call 911?
Financial obligations been met?	Yes	

Once the patient has arrived home, it is important to realize that the family and those serving as caregivers may have difficulty in perceiving how much care the patient will need. The caregivers will also need emotional support as they deal with the transition and challenges caring for a patient entails. No one caregiver can give care 24 hours a day, 7 days a week. In cases where the patient is too debilitated to leave home on their own, they need someone who can help them out in the case of a fire. However, through it all, remember: providing care, time and love are the only gifts you can give your loved one, and the only gifts he or she will want.

Bedside Story

Hilda felt the hospital was no place to live or die. She wanted to go home. Her family agreed. Fortunately, we found a nurse and doctor who believed in the benefits of a hospice program. This program, for terminally ill patients, provides support services emphasizing comfort and care rather than cures.

We were so thankful when Hilda was discharged to hospice on Labor Day. I was amazed that we were able to take her home on a holiday and have the necessary support and supplies provided that day. We had a hospital bed set up in her living room and were provided with the necessary lifts, wheelchairs and supplies. Hospice was wonderful throughout Hilda's stay at home, providing intermittent nursing care and support.

Hilda needed twenty-four hour nursing care. What we did not anticipate was that no insurance policy covers this type of care, which is very expensive and costs between $6,000 and $10,000 a month. By pooling all of Hilda's resources with those of family members, we were able to provide her with this level of care.

I took care of Hilda during the first week she was at home and spent that time arranging for the proper care. There are a number of agencies that provide twenty-four hour in-home care. One of the best is *Comfort Keepers*. Julie, the owner, personally interviewed Hilda, assessed the home for what was needed, and continually monitored the situation.

Hilda's coming home provided us with an opportunity to be really creative, trying to make the problem-solving process fun and dynamic. Since Hilda lived in an upstairs apartment, we hired day workers to help lift her, on the wheelchair, down the stairs. The workers were wonderful and anxious to help Hilda. This provided a way for her to go out.

Once we had figured a way for Hilda to go out, we were surprised at how accommodating movie theatres, restaurants and other venues were to a person in a wheelchair. Mom's cooking club brought parties to her bedside where everyone brought their own plates, food, and drink.

*Key Points

- Plan for discharge before the event occurs.

- Be creative and look at alternatives that may not have been considered by others.

- Look at discharge as an adventure, and a way to have your loved one in his or her own environment.

- Have resources ready and available.

- Don't be afraid to call healthcare persons for questions and concerns.

- Do everything you can to decrease frustrations on the day of discharge. Help your loved one to feel that this is a seamless transition.

- Have a telephone close by that cannot be dropped.

Notes

_____

_____

_____

_____

_____

_____

_____

_____

_____

_____

_____

_____

_____

_____

_____

_____

Dealings With Feelings: Emotional Responses to Illness

The experts give us theories to
Soften what we must go through.
They tell us what we all will face,
Before we leave this earthly place.

And this we hope describes our life,
We substituted peace for strife.
Protected nature's precious gifts,
And down-cast spirits did uplift.

Our time and wealth and love we shared,
We offered hope and showed we cared.
Debased no person, gender, race
And leave the world a better place.

CHAPTER 10
Dealings With Feelings: Emotional Responses to Illness

Although all the information in this book should be of value to you, this chapter is particularly important because it deals with those feelings that occur when your loved one becomes ill. Freud's Theory of Regression and Maslow's Hierarchy of Needs will help explain the behavior of the patient, while Elisabeth Kubler-Ross identifies the stages of loss that both patient and caregiver will experience if the illness of the patient is terminal. Summarizing these theories will help to explain the feelings that occur for both the caregiver and the patient. These feelings are normal, and once understood, can be dealt with through understanding and patience.

Freud's Theory of Regression

Often a patient will respond to illness by regressing, where they adopt childlike behaviors. If the patient for whom you are providing care is young, he or she may start sucking their thumb again or may wet the bed. However, if the patient is a spouse, parent, or older friend, who is used to being seen as strong and self-reliant, the change might be even more disconcerting. The adult may whine, pout, and even throw mini-tantrums. In either case, you will find that you must maintain your role as the adult, showing that you can help meet the patient's needs and allay his or her fears.

Maslow's Hierarchy of Needs

In order to understand the theory behind the behaviors, we look to Abraham Maslow's Hierarchy of Needs.

Maslow tells us that each level of need must be met or fulfilled before a person is ready to move up to the next need level. The first set of needs that must be met for the patient are basic physiological ones: oxygen, water, food, and elimination.

Self-Actualization
Self Development
Ego/Self-Esteem Needs
Recognition and Status
Social Needs
Belongingness and Love
Safety Needs
Security and Protection
Physiologic Needs
Hunger, Thirst, Oxygen, Food and Elimination

Once these needs have been met, safety concerns will become the focus. "Will I fall out of bed?" "How can I call for help?" "Will anybody respond if I need help?" "Who will bring my bedpan?" If the patient is in the hospital or another type of care facility where a nursing staff is present, the answers are relatively simple. The hospital staff will meet both the physiological and safety needs. However, if the patient is being discharged home, meeting both sets of these needs becomes much more complicated. The anxiety that the patient feels must be relieved by the actions and words of the caregiver. The caregiver must be able to answer the patient's concerns and fears with assured, concrete information.

Once the physiological and safety needs have been satisfied, Maslow identifies the third level of needs: Love and Belonging. For the patient, this means that friends and family members need to visit and demonstrate their support and love for the patient. Having your loved one surrounded by those who love him can greatly assist the patient in promoting recovery.

When Maslow's bottom three levels of needs have been satisfied and as the patient begins to feel better and/or adapt to his/her new situation, then the self-esteem, cognitive and aesthetic needs can be addressed. This is the time when you reintroduce some of the activities that the patient enjoyed before the illness in which they can once again participate actively. Depending on their interests, this can be going to a movie, dining out, attending a play or art gallery or simply reading or being read to- whatever will help to stimulate the brain, satisfying mental and emotional needs. In addition, any activities that strengthen the body should also be encouraged. Physical therapy and the subsequent increased mobility a patient will experience add to a sense of independence and competence, whether it is the patient's newly developed ability to feed himself or herself or the few steps a patient can take using a walker.

Using Maslow's theory, a caregiver can better understand where to focus his or her energy. There is no sense in trying to create activities to increase a patient's sense of competence when the patient is consumed with worry over who will be there to help them go to the bathroom at night.

Kubler-Ross' Stages of Grief

Elisabeth Kubler-Ross helped explain the continuum of grief when faced with impending death by isolating and identifying five stages that both the patient and caregivers will endure. By dividing the grief process into stages, Kubler-Ross helped the grief-stricken person understand that these experiences and emotions are normal. Some people will quickly progress through all the phases, while others appear to get "stuck" in a particular phase. It is important to understand that family members, friends, and caregivers may be in a different phase than the patient. For example, the patient may have accepted the reality of death, but the family is in denial, refusing to admit the possibility that their loved one may die.

Briefly, the stages of grief as identified by Elisabeth Kubler-Ross are outlined below.

1. Shock and Denial- the reality of death or impending death has not yet hit, and there is the feeling that this illness

or condition cannot be real. There is the thought, "No, this can't be happening to me." This is a normal reaction to protect oneself from facing reality.

2. Anger- the patient or grief-stricken person often lashes out at the family, friends, the doctors, hospital staff and/or world in general. There is the thought of "Why me?" Many people will also experience guilt or fear during this stage.

3. Bargaining- in this stage, the patient or bereaved person attempts to change reality by making agreements with God, their loved ones, and is usually the beginning of acceptance. You may hear statements such as, "I want to live until the wedding," or "I'll pray every day if this goes away."

4. Depression- depression occurs as a reaction to the changed way of life created by the illness. The patient and the caregiver feel intensely sad, hopeless and helpless. The patient may review his or her life and may feel despair.

5. Acceptance- acceptance comes when there is a resolution of feelings about impending death. The patient is neither happy nor sad and is ready to let go. The patient may actually try to protect or comfort those that he or she leaves behind.

While much of the attention in this chapter has been focused upon the patient, it is also important to recognize the needs of the caregiver. Often, the caregivers spend too much time focusing upon how the suffering and death of their loved one impacts their own life. This normal, natural reaction affects the ability to be a necessary support to the patient. Moreover, the caregivers undergo tremendous stress as they struggle with watching their loved one die. The caregivers also need positive love and support as they struggle with their own sense of loss, trying to remember that we must be thankful for the time that we have had with our loved one, not regretting the time we will miss.

Bedside Story

Members of our family experienced different reactions to Hilda's illness at different times. Our levels of anger at what was happening to her and feelings of loss occurred in isolation from one another. This was good for us, as we were able to give each other fresh perspectives. My understanding of some of the psychological principles helped me understand some of the feelings I was experiencing and allowed me to take help and comfort from my family and friends when I needed support.

Hilda surprised us by being quite amenable to being taken care of by others. This was surprising for a woman who had always been fiercely independent. Hilda seemed to enjoy the dependent role. My sisters and I discussed this behavior and concluded that this may have been the first time in her life that she had been cared for in such a way. She was, in a way, experiencing what a child does- total care and nurturing.

There were times when Hilda seemed ready to fight. She was such a trooper. She held her head high, in her wheelchair and even though she was paralyzed, traveled places she once vigorously walked.

While Hilda did not have a terminal illness, she continued to deteriorate. One day, she asked to speak to each of us separately. She said she did not want to continue to live this way and wanted to know how we would feel if she gave up. We each responded that we would fully support her in whatever she wanted to do. We told her that we loved her, and that if she wanted to go on with life, we would make it happen to the best of our ability. If, however, she was really tired and wanted to let go, we would support her decision. Hilda told us she was so relieved that we felt this way. She said she wanted to let go but didn't know how we felt. It seemed she was hanging on for us. Within days, Hilda gradually became less responsive, then passed away. How interesting that she was ready to accept her death before we were.

*Key Points

- There are no textbook phrases or answers to how anyone feels in the situation when their loved one becomes ill.

- Understanding some of the psychological dynamics can make the horrible feel more predictable and normal.

- Even if you are the fiercely independent type, let others help you. It lets them do something loving for you.

- Expressing your feelings by writing can be therapeutic. You don't need to write for anyone else's eyes, but the writing will help you express what is happening to you.

Notes

Epilogue

One day Hilda called and asked to speak to each of us separately. She asked us if it was all right with us for her to "let go", that she really didn't want to live this way. Each of us, in our own way, gave our mother the same answer. "We will support whatever decision you make. If you want to live, we will do whatever you desire to make your life joyful and productive. If you want to die, we will support your wishes and honor your request." Our mother broke into tears and said she was so relieved that we felt that way and thankful we were together.

Within a few days, on February 13, 2002, at 12:45 p.m., we received "THE CALL". One of Hilda's wonderful caregivers, Christina, called in tears to say that Hilda had stopped breathing. This was fitting, as Christina had been encouraged by Hilda to become a nurse. Another caregiver, Jennifer, came to be with Hilda when she heard the news.

Family and friends were called and invited to be with her at her home before she was taken away. We found it was important to let immediate relatives and close friends know right away, to give them the choice of coming to the home. Hilda's children, grandchildren, great-grandchildren, stepmother, sister, and her wonderful friend Doris rushed to be by her side.

There was discussion about whether to call this person or that. Should we disturb them at work? Should we wait? I can answer that emphatically by saying, "CALL NOW; CALL FAST" and give the person a choice. All of us who came were very thankful that we were there.

We did something unusual, and asked that she be picked up by the Neptune Society in a few hours. As a result, we had the opportunity to "hang out" with Hilda for hours after she passed away. This was a wonderful experience as we gathered around her, lit a candle, and talked about the wonderful influence Hilda had on all of our lives.

We all held hands around Hilda's bed, as Linda led us in a prayer that sealed our love for Hilda and one another.

There was an amazing change that occurred with Hilda's face during the time we were with her. Initially we had to close her eyes and she seemed very stiff. After a few hours, her mouth turned into a smile and her whole countenance relaxed.

For our family, this had been the worst of times, and the best of times. Hilda's illness brought us together on a daily basis and created a closeness that the three of us now have that we never had experienced before. Our mother had the chance to tell us how much she loved us, and we too had the opportunity to share our love for her. Hilda's brother, Eric, and his wife, Coral, came from halfway around the world to see Hilda, and we had the chance to get to see and know our uncle and aunt better.

As Hilda wanted to be cremated, we followed her wishes, and sailed out to sea to deliver her ashes to her beloved ocean. Hilda's nephew and niece escorted us on their boat for the journey out to sea. The day was perfect; the sky was blue, and we gathered as a united family to put her out to sea to surf her final and endless wave.

On Hilda's birthday, July 5, 2002, we met at her favorite beach, Diver's Cove, and the three of us swam out in the waves for a memorial swim in her honor. Her friends and other family watched from the shore as we said our final goodbye.

Our hope is that you never have to use the information in this book, but should you need the resource, our desire is that you have the necessary tools to advocate effectively and successfully for your loved one.

Our family is thankful for the opportunity to spread the word and share our experiences. You may reach us on Hilda's Website, www.helpinghilda.com. We invite you to share your experiences.

With Love,

Linda Cooper
Trish Billings
Terry Rudd

An Interview with Hilda's Daughters

Linda - I am 55 and the eldest daughter. I've lived in Laguna Beach, California for 30 years and have a 14-year-old daughter, Azure Rose. My main life work has been as a landscape designer and builder. I currently spend my time between Laguna and Sedona, Arizona while working on producing a book showing my garden creations and crystal creations as a means for sharing my spiritual wisdom.

Trish – I am 53, the middle child and have been married to my husband, John, for 29 years. I have 3 grown children, Shaylor, an air force fighter pilot, Ariane, a senior at Princeton Univ, and John, a freshman at UC Santa Barbara. I have a bookkeeping business that I operate out of my home office in Mission Beach, California. My passions, body-surfing and various sports, are a legacy from my mom, Hilda.

Terry – I am 50 years old and the baby of the family. I have three grown children: Sharon Brown, a registered nurse, Karen Genco, a physician's assistant, and Erin Rudd, who has her master's in clinical psychology. My two grandchildren, Tyler and Sydney Brown give me pure joy. I have been a registered nurse for 29 years with an emphasis in Critical Care Nursing and Education. In addition to my full-time teaching at the local community college, I have a thriving healthcare educational business called Flex Ed.

Why was it important to get this book written?

Terry: I truly wanted to write the book to help others who have hospitalized loved ones. If I, as an R.N., missed important details, what happens to persons who do not have the frame of reference and knowledge that I have? If the book helps one person, I will be happy. In writing the book, I have sent rough drafts to friends and family who needed the information. Every person said the information was essential for understanding and helping advocate for their hospitalized family member. I also wanted everyone to know what a remarkable woman our mother was.

Trish: It was important to get this book written because there is a problem with our health system today. We were brought up to believe that our doctors knew everything and could fix everything and that we should hand over our loved ones to their care. Many factors, including a nursing shortage, make it difficult for the hospital staff to pay attention in the way that we have come to expect.

I don't believe that it is possible any longer for us as individuals to relinquish so much control and expect good results. I felt that we just didn't know enough to help Mom out. Different people kept telling us different things. We didn't know enough to make the right decisions or give her the proper care. As the caregivers for our loved ones, everyone must have the knowledge that this book contains so that what happened to our mother doesn't happen to your loved one.

Linda: This book needed to be written to assist others in helping themselves and their family members through physical, mental and emotional challenges - to assist others in understanding the nature of being supportive of their loved ones and helping them to get through the arduous process of healing in a hospital.

Could you briefly describe your mother?

Linda: Hilda was very caring and generous of spirit. She was interested in people and their stories and interested in sharing her stories with others. She was a woman of high vitality, interested in life and adventure on all levels.

Trish: Mom was adventurous, always positive, always looking for the good in people and she was fun to be around. She left us to live our own lives. She didn't interfere. She had her own life and activities to keep her busy and interested in living, and she really didn't need us there to be part of it. She was very independent.

Terry: My mother lived a remarkable life. She was a trailblazer for her time and truly helped many people in her life. My mother had friends who were from all walks of life and of many different ages. She would make a stranger a friend in a heartbeat.

Can you tell us a little bit about your mother's life?

Trish: Mom grew up in South Africa, where she and her brother were children of divorced parents at a time when parents didn't get divorced. There was a lot of shame connected to this. She was put into a Catholic convent where she was the only Jewish girl, and when her father came to visit or take her away from the convent, there wasn't much love involved in the process. From that beginning, she went to nursing school and became a fantastic nurse. She only liked the challenging-type nursing jobs. She liked working with people, particularly kids, and that was exhibited in her emergency room work, her free clinic work, and her student health work. She was a no-nonsense nurse, very pragmatic, and often knew more than the doctors did about her specialty. She took her first trip when I was about 16 years old. She went to Hawaii with only a backpack and had the most marvelous time. From then on, she took one trip a year and ended up traveling to nearly 100 countries around the world during her life. On each trip, she tried to take full advantage of everything that the country had to offer. She had so many friends, she didn't know what to do with them all. Everyone in Laguna Beach wanted to be friends with Hilda. With her children, she was a "hands-off granny". She helped us when she could, but she rarely told us how to do it. She adored her grandchildren, and her favorite thing was to teach them how to go swimming in the ocean past the waves. She taught me to surf and gave me a lifelong love for the ocean. She encouraged me to be an independent woman, to stand up for myself, and she helped me to understand that I could achieve whatever I wanted to.

Terry: My mother was a very hard worker. She always juggled work with family and friends. She was the working mom who was also the Girl Scout leader. When we were growing up, often she was the only mother that I knew that worked. As a nurse, she gave wonderful care to her patients. She once said that she had been a nurse for 50 years and never had a bad day of work.

Linda: My mother's life was full of hard work and difficulty, especially early on. Her younger life was one of being abandoned by her parents. At a young age, she wanted to become a nurse, so she really went against what was the mainstream in those days. She really enjoyed serving and caring for others. She held the energy of an open heart for many people in her life, and she was a good provider as a mother, a friend, and as a working partner.

Hilda was loved by her associates at work, as well as the patients who came into the university health center. People loved her stories and the energy she gave. She had the ability to be a light to people on the journey of life. Hilda particularly loved babies. So she was really kind of what I would call a "sparkle farkle".

Hilda's thirst for knowledge was also incredible. She was always reading. She loved history and studied, read, and watched documentaries about the past. Hilda was very involved in the arts, being the first to see whatever play or movie or art form was current. She never lost her desire to learn. She was always open to "the new" and stayed connected to young people. She also really enjoyed adventures. She was always exploring new territories. Her love for the ocean was great. Each time I go to ocean, she is with me. She was quite an amazing person.

It is tragic that Hilda died at 82, but hadn't she already led a full life?

Linda: Yes, she had lived an extremely full life. Her earlier life was filled with difficulties, but her later life was filled with adventure and fun. So in that respect, she had truly mastered her challenges and had transformed them into play, which for me is the journey of everybody's life. Through her careful monitoring of her income, she was able to live a free, adventurous life. She never expected anyone to take care of her. She was self sufficient, and assumed total responsibility for herself, an admirable quality. She was amazing and yet, I don't think she was necessarily finished.

Terry: Hilda lived a full life every day she lived. She was fiercely independent and made a great effort not to be a burden on others. At 82, she continued to swim in the ocean every day, develop new friendships, and become an integral part of the lives of her children, grandchildren and great-grandchildren. I could easily have seen her live to 100 with many productive years in between.

Trish: Oh, my gosh, no. Every moment, every minute had the expectation of 20 more years in it.

What do you think is Hilda's legacy?

Terry: Hilda's legacy is that you live life to the fullest and forge ahead, despite obstacles.

Linda: Her legacy was her zest for life, her willingness for adventure, her undying fortitude in continuing to live her passion, and her assuming personal responsibility at all times.

Trish: Mom's legacy is to be intrepid, to not be afraid to try anything and to find the positive in everything.

What was the effect of her illness on you and your family?

Trish: The joy of seeing her move her legs immediately after the surgery was unbelievably euphoric. I was thrilled; I was ecstatic. I was thankful. When I heard that she had lost sensation, I was devastated. I couldn't believe that my indefatigable mom, this woman, who survived so many things and had such a positive attitude, who suddenly would never be able to walk again, sent me to the depths of despair. When she became so weak that she couldn't feed herself, I couldn't believe it. I had never seen her in a position where she couldn't take care of herself. I kept waiting for her to get better. I just knew she would. And when she didn't and couldn't, I could barely even think about it. My family couldn't believe it either. They kept waiting to hear from me that she was getting better.

Linda: Her illness was a unifying force that brought my sisters and me closer together. We rallied around her and all assisted her in her transition and by so doing, we unified our family unit. Another result of her illness is that it has brought all three sisters to a new level of awareness of our relationships to each other and our need to be of service to humanity. It has helped us focus on working creatively together to write this book. Her illness really has catalyzed our life work.

Terry: Hilda's illness was the best of times and the worst of times for our family. Her illness brought my sisters and me closer together, as we had never been before in our lives. We were able to rally around the same cause and utilize our individual talents to help our mom. Her illness gave us a chance to let her know how we felt about her and also gave her and us the opportunity to see all the friends and family that truly cared about her. Hilda's illness was also the worst of times for us, as the unfortunate paralysis left our mother completely dependent upon others for most of her needs. This dependence was new for Hilda, and it really upset her.

What was your role in your mother's care?

Terry: I essentially became her case manager and caretaker. I handled all the medical aspects. I was the interpreter for others in the family who didn't understand what was going on and was often the person to relay information to the medical team.

Linda: My role in her care was spiritual, meaning I was to show up, hold her hand and be there for her. My job was to surround her with a positive force, using her energy and mine, so that she wouldn't have fear.

Trish: My role was to take care of the financial aspects of her life for which she had never needed any help before. It was also to talk to her and see to her needs from a pragmatic point of view. When I came to visit, instead of talking about her care, we talked more about what she wanted for the rest of her life, what her wishes were, and how we could help her to achieve them.

If you could rewind time, what would you do differently?

Trish: I would have made sure one of us never left her side. I would have made sure that there was immediate action taken the moment she became distressed at the loss of feeling. I would have slept by her bedside and made sure that all her needs had been taken care of. If I had known who to call and who could help her, I would have pursued them with a vengeance. What was missing in Mom's care was a personal advocate who had nothing to do but take care of her, and I would gladly have been that person. I wish I had known that it was so necessary.

Terry: I would have been with her when she lost sensation and became paralyzed. I believe if I had been there, the medical team would have acted in a timelier manner, which might have prevented her paralysis. By the time I got the news, it was too late. I have no regrets for the love and caring we gave our mother during her illness. As a family, I think we were great.

Linda – It's always difficult to answer that type of question. Hilda had an exquisite life and I believe everything is divinely orchestrated and that everything happens the way it does for a reason.

What advice would you give someone who has just been admitted to the hospital?

Linda: My advice would be only to enter the hospital if you absolutely have to. Do everything in your power to stay calm and be very clear about what you want to accomplish when entering the hospital. Don't be afraid to ask questions and communicate your desires. Stay focused on health and healing. Love yourself throughout the experience. Release your fears and keep your heart open, knowing that you will be well taken care of, provided for, and will come through this with ease and grace.

Trish: Read our book. Do what it says. Don't be afraid to

ask questions. Don't be afraid to demand action, and stay by your loved one's side no matter what any hospital staff member might say. Bring a good book.

Terry: Ask someone to stay with you and decipher what is going on. Do not be afraid to ask questions and be assertive if you feel someone or something is needed for your loved one's care. Listen to your intuition and act upon it. If the care you are getting is not what you think it should be, communicate your thoughts and feelings immediately with the medical team. Do not be afraid to repeat yourself in an assertive manner.

APPENDICES

Personal Data

Name

_____

Address

_____

Telephone

_____

Work Phone

_____

Occupation

_____

Health Plan Name

_____

Health Plan Number

_____

Health Plan Phone

_____

Emergency Contact Name

_____

Emergency Contact Phone

_____

Name and Phone Number of Key Individuals (family, friends, significant others)

Person's Name	Relationship	Telephone (area code)

Physician(s) Name and Phone Number

Physician Name	Specialty	Telephone (area code)

Medical History: Previous Illnesses, Hospitalizations, and Surgeries

Family History

Mother

_____

Father

_____

Brother(s)

_____

Sister(s)

_____

Previous Illnesses and Operations	Year Diagnosed	Current Status Continues or Resolved

Hospitalization Reason	Date	Place	Length of Stay

Surgery Reason	Date	Place

Recent Travel _____

Exposure to someone with a communicable disease?_____

_____

Drug or Food Allergy Or Sensitivity_____

Drug or Food Name	Reaction

Current Medication

Medication Name	Dosage	Times per Day	Last Dose Taken

Appendix B: Chapter 2
Advanced Directive Card

Advanced Directive Card

Name: _____

I have an Advanced Directive on File at:

_____

Call _____ for a copy.

Appendix C: Chapter 3
Additional Physicians

Specialist	Area of Responsibility
Cardiovascular Surgeon	Surgical treatment of the heart and blood vessels.
Dermatologist	Skin disorders.
Emergency Physician	Emergency treatment of conditions caused by trauma or sudden illness.
Gerontologist	Diseases of the elderly.
Hematologist	Blood disorders.
Hospitalist	Cares for patient only while in the hospital.
Immunologist	Allergic disorders and the management of the body's immune system.
Neurosurgeon	Surgical treatment of the central nervous system and disorders.
Obstetrician	Pregnant women and the fetus.
Ophthalmologist	Medical and surgical treatment of eye disorders.
Orthopedist, Orthopod	Medical and surgical treatment of the bones, muscles and joints.
Otolaryngologist, ENT	Medical and surgical treatment of the ears, nose and throat.
Pathologist	Diagnosis of diseases by analyzing cells obtained at biopsy or autopsy.
Pediatrician	Care and treatment of children.
Plastic surgeon	Surgery for alteration, replacement, and restoration of body structures due to a defect or for cosmetic reasons.
Podiatrist	Disorders and surgeries of the feet.
Proctologist	Colon, rectum, and anus.
Psychiatrist	Mental, emotional and behavioral disorders.
Rheumatologist	Treatment of joint and muscle disorders.

Appendix D: Chapter 3
Communication Logs

Patient Name:_____

Lead Advocate: _____

Other Advocate: _____

Allergies: _____

Physicians to See Patient

Physician	Specialty	Date Seen	Communication

Other Persons to See Patient

Person	Specialty	Date Seen	Communication

Patient Concerns

Date	Concern	Person Notified	Communication	Date Resolved

Advocate Concerns

Date	Concern	Person Notified	Communication	Date Resolved

Appendix E: Chapter 4
Additional Abbreviations

ABBREVIATION	MEANING
ABO	A system of classifying blood groups. Used for blood typing.
ACE	Angiotensin converting enzyme A classification of drugs that helps with blood pressure and congestive heart failure.
ACTH	Adrenocorticotropic hormone, corticotropin Blood levels checked to see if there is a deficiency.
ADH	Antidiuretic hormone May measure this lab level to see if there is a deficiency in the hormone.
ad lib	As desired
AIDS	Acquired Immunodeficiency Syndrome
ALT	Alanine aminotransferase (formerly SGPT)
AST	Aspartate aminotransferase (formerly SGOT)
ANA	Antinuclear antibody
AP	Anteroposterior Describes anatomical positioning, usually in an x-ray.
A&P	Anterior and posterior Describes anatomical positioning, usually in an x-ray.
AQ	Water, usually refers to a solution that is watery.
ARDS	Adult respiratory distress syndrome is a severe respiratory disturbance that has many causes. Most often, the patient is put on a ventilator (breathing machine) to try and resolve the problem.
ASHD	Atherosclerotic heart disease. A general term to describe heart disease where the arteries harden. This can result in a heart attack.
BLS	Basic life support. Includes CPR or basic resuscitation when the person stops breathing.
BMR	Basal metabolic rate. A determination of an individual's metabolic rate to help determine caloric needs.

ABBREVIATION	MEANING
BPH	Benign prostatic hypertrophy. An enlargement of the prostate gland that is not cancer.
bpm	Beats per minute. Used in referring to heart rate or pulse.
BSA	Body surface area. A calculation derived from the person's height and weight. Is utilized to determine optimum drug dosages and caloric intake.
BX	Biopsy. A body tissue sample is taken to determine how the cells look. A biopsy is often done to help diagnose cancer.
C	Celsius, centigrade. A way to measure body temperature. Some facilities use Celsius or centigrade rather than Fahrenheit. 98.6 F is equal to 37 C.
CAD	Coronary artery disease. A general term for blockage of the arteries that supplies the heart muscle. Blockage of these arteries is the cause of a heart attack.
caps	Capsules. Medications are supplied in capsules.
CCU	Coronary care unit. The place in the hospital where cardiac or heart patients are housed in a critical setting.
CEA	Carcinoembryonic antigen. A blood test to help diagnose cancer and see the effects of cancer treatment.
CK, CPK	Creatine kinase. A blood enzyme test to see if there is damage to the heart muscle.
Cl	Chloride, chlorine. A blood test.
CLL	Chronic lymphocytic leukemia. A classification of leukemia.
cm	Centimeter. A unit of measure. There are 2.2 cm to an inch. Most small measurements in the hospital are done using a centimeter ruler.
CO	Carbon monoxide, cardiac output. Carbon monoxide levels are blood levels that may be checked. The cardiac output is a calculation done either by ultrasound or by a computer to see how well the heart is contracting.

ABBREVIATION	MEANING
CO2	Carbon dioxide. A lab test done either with a venous blood sample (a base) or an arterial blood sample (an acid) to determine the patient's acid base status.
CPR	Cardiopulmonary resuscitation, and a part of basic life support when the patient has stopped breathing or the heart has stopped.
C&S	Culture and sensitivity. This blood test is done to identify bacteria (culture) and determine which antibiotic is best (sensitivity)
CSF	Cerebrospinal fluid. This is fluid taken from the spinal column to check for bleeding or bacteria. This fluid is obtained through a procedure called a spinal tap or lumbar puncture.
CTS	Carpal tunnel syndrome. A disorder on the hands often caused from repetitive stress to the area.
DC	Discharge or discontinue.
DIC	Disseminated intravascular coagulation. A serious, usually life-threatening situation with many causes that results in a combination of clotting in the small vessels of the body and bleeding everywhere else.
DIFF, diff	Differential blood count. This blood test separates the different types of white blood cells to help determine the possible cause of an infection.
DO	Doctor of osteopathy. A physician who has medical training as an M.D. and also has increased training in muscle and tissue manipulation.
DPT	Diphtheria, pertussis, and tetanus (toxoids/vaccine). A vaccine.
D/W	Dextrose in water. A common I.V. solution that is sugar water. A full liter only contains 200 calories and is sometimes the only nourishment a patient may receive.
EEG	Electroencephalogram. This test to check the electrical activity of the brain, is useful for diagnosing seizures. This is sometimes the test that is used to determine if someone is brain dead.

ABBREVIATION	MEANING
EMG	Electromyogram. A test to see how the muscles respond to electrical stimulation.
ENT	Ear, nose, and throat. A medical specialty.
ESR	Erythrocyte sedimentation rate. A blood test that may indicate inflammation or tissue injury.
F	Fahrenheit. A way to measure temperature. Normal body temperature is 98.6 degrees. The equivalent for centigrade is 37 degrees.
FSH	Follicle-stimulating hormone. A blood test to check the hormone level.
ft	Foot, feet (measure)
FUO	Fever of undetermined origin. Diagnosis used until the cause of a fever is determined.
GFR	Glomerular filtration rate. A determination of how the kidneys are filtering the blood.
GI	Gastrointestinal. Includes structures from the mouth, stomach, small intestines and large intestine.
gr	Grain. An old unit of measure. Drugs are sometimes ordered in grains.
gt, gtt	Drop, drops. Usually the abbreviation for eye or ear drops.
GTT	Glucose tolerance test. A test to determine a person's ability to metabolize glucose. A sweet syrupy substance is given and blood sugars are tested regularly (hourly) up to 5 hours to check for the possibility of diabetes.
GU	Genitourinary. Body system that includes the kidneys, the tubes that lead to the bladder (ureters), and the bladder and tube that go from the bladder to the outside of the body (urethra). Also includes the genital area.
GYN, gyn	Gynecology. Specialty that covers female reproductive system.
HCG	Human chorionic gonadotropin. A hormone level.

ABBREVIATION	MEANING
HCL	Hydrochloric acid, hydrochloride. A blood test.
HCO3	Bicarbonate. A base that can be tested in the arterial or venous blood.
HDL	High-density lipoprotein. A blood test that is part of the cholesterol panel.
HDN	Hemolytic disease of the newborn.
Hg	Mercury. Many measurements are calculated in millimeters of mercury such as blood pressure and cardiac output calculations.
HGH	Human growth hormone
IABP	Intra-aortic balloon pump. A device used to help the severely compromised heart rest. This is an invasive procedure where the device is placed in a large artery (ascending aorta) and has a balloon that is inflated to help deliver oxygenated blood to the heart.
IgA, IgD, IgE, IgG	Immunoglobulins to help determine a patient's level of immunity.
IHSS	Idiopathic hypertrophic subaortic stenosis
inf	Inferior. An anatomical location.
inj	Inject
IPPB	Intermittent positive-pressure breathing. A breathing treatment usually given by the respiratory therapy department that contains a drug, given by inhalation, that helps open up the airway or loosen secretions.
IUD	Intrauterine device. A device placed in the cervix of the uterus to help prevent pregnancy.
I.V.	Intravenous. Solutions that are placed into a vein to deliver fluid and/or drugs.
IVP	Intravenous pyelogram. An x-ray exam that looks at the kidneys, ureters (tubes from kidney to bladder), and bladder, after the injection of an iodine-based dye.
JRA	Juvenile rheumatoid arthritis
kcal	Kilocalorie (food calorie).

ABBREVIATION	MEANING
kg	Kilogram. A measure of weight. Some facilities weigh patients in pounds and others in Kg. There are 2.2 pounds in 1 kilogram.
KUB	Kidneys, ureters, and bladder. An x-ray exam.
L	Liter. A liquid unit of measure. I.V. solutions are usually hung in liters, which is about the same as a pint.
lat	Lateral. Means the side. The patient may be asked to lie on the left lateral side, or the left side.
lb	Pound
LBBB	Left bundle branch block. An electrical abnormality of the heart that will show on the EKG.
LDH	Lactate dehydrogenase. A blood enzyme test to determine damage to the liver or heart.
LDL	Low-density lipoprotein. A blood test that is part of the cholesterol assessment.
LE	Lupus erythematosus, a chronic inflammatory disease.
LH	Luteinizing hormone. This is secreted by the pituitary gland in the brain to determine sex hormone production.
lt	Left
LUQ	Left upper quadrant. An anatomical location on the stomach.
LV	Left ventricle. The left lower chamber of the heart.
m	Meter, minim. Meter is a measure of length. Minim is a liquid measure that is very small.
MD	Medical Doctor
mm	Millimeter. A unit of measure to determine length. Millimeters are very small and sometimes used to measure tumor size.
MS	Multiple sclerosis, morphine sulfate
MUGA	Multigated acquisition (scanning)
NaCl	Sodium chloride. Same as normal saline. A common I.V. solution and irrigating solution.

ABBREVIATION	MEANING
Ob-GYN	Obstetrics and gynecology. A medical specialty dealing with female disorders and reproduction.
oz	Ounce
PaCO2	Partial pressure of carbon dioxide in arterial blood. The normal range is 35-45.
PaO2	Partial pressure of oxygen in arterial blood. The normal range is 80-100.
Pap	Papanicolaou smear. Taken from the vagina or cervix to determine if there are cells that may be precancerous or cancerous.
PCO2	Partial pressure of carbon dioxide. Taken from arterial blood. Normal range is 35-45.
PO2	Partial pressure of oxygen. Taken from arterial blood. Normal range is 80-100.
peds	Pediatrics. A medical specialty that deals with children.
Perrla	Pupils equal, round, react to light and accommodation. A light is shone in the eyes to check the status of the neurological system.
pH	Hydrogen ion concentration. This test indicates whether the person is in a state of acidosis or alkalosis. Normal range is 7.35 – 7.45.
PID	Pelvic inflammatory disease.
PKU	Phenylketonuria. A newborn screening test to check for the lack of an enzyme that metabolizes amino acids.
PMS	Premenstrual syndrome
PPD	Purified protein derivative (of tuberculin). An injection given in the inside of the forearm to see if the person has antibodies to or has tuberculosis. A positive PPD does not necessarily mean the person has tuberculosis.

ABBREVIATION	MEANING
PTCA	Percutaneous transluminal coronary angioplasty. This procedure is used to treat blockage of the coronary arteries that causes a heart attack. A catheter with a small balloon on the end is threaded through an artery in the groin to the arteries of the heart. The catheter is threaded to the area of blockage and the balloon is inflated many times to compress the blockage against the walls of the artery.
PTH	Parathyroid hormone. Checks levels from the gland located behind the thyroid. Responsible for calcium and phosphorus production.
PVC	Premature ventricular contraction. An irregular early beat from the lower chambers of the heart.
RA	Rheumatoid arthritis
RF	Rheumatic fever, rheumatoid factor
Rh pos. or neg	Rhesus factor positive or negative
SBE	Subacute bacterial endocarditis. A bacterial infection that produces growths on the cells lining the heart wall.
sed rate	Erythrocyte sedimentation rate. A blood test that may indicate inflammation or tissue injury.
SGOT	Serum glutamic-oxalacetic transaminase (see AST). An enzyme to check for damage to the liver.
SGPT	An enzyme to check for damage to the liver.
SIDS	Sudden infant death syndrome.
SLE	Systemic lupus erythematosus, an inflammatory disease of the blood, with features including fever, weakness, fatigability, joint pains and skin lesions on the face, neck or arms
STD	Sexually transmitted disease
T&A	Tonsillectomy and adenoidectomy
TIA	Transient ischemic attack. Sometimes called a temporary stroke, with the same symptoms of a stroke, but they go away. When a TIA occurs, this is often a warning sign to do diagnostic testing to prevent an actual stroke.

ABBREVIATION	MEANING
TPR	Temperature, pulse, respirations. Part of the vital signs.
tsp	Teaspoon
URI	Upper respiratory infection. An infection in the lungs.
VDRL	Venereal Disease Research Laboratory (test for syphilis).
Vfib, VF	Ventricular fibrillation. An abnormal heart rhythm that must be treated by electrical shock.
VT	Ventricular tachycardia. An abnormal heart rhythm that may be treated with drugs or electrical shock.
UTI	Urinary tract infection. May be an infection of the bladder or kidneys.

Appendix F: Chapter 6
Additional Lab Values

Lab Value	Normal Ranges	Significance	What to ask? And Consider
Acetone, Ketone Bodies	Acetone – negative, ketones 0.5-4 mg/dl	The test may be done to check for diabetes or malnutrition.	Is the patient losing fat because of malnutrition?
Alcohol	negative	Generally, an alcohol level of greater than 0.1 or 100 mg/dl is an indication of alcohol intoxication.	Why might the level be positive?
Ammonia	15-45 mcg/dl	Ammonia is a by-product of protein metabolism. When there are problems with the liver, the level may exhibit temporary elevation.	A low protein diet may aid in decreasing the ammonia level.
Amylase	60 – 160 U/dl or 30-170 U/l	Often done to diagnose pancreatitis. May also be increased with abdominal surgery, diabetes, and alcoholic intoxication.	Patients with increased amylase should control alcohol intake and increase protein and carbohydrates in the diet.

Lab Value	Normal Ranges	Significance	What to ask? And Consider
Bilirubin Prehepatic, unconjugated, and free-indirect reacting are the same.	Prehepatic 0.1 – 1.0 mg/dl	This is a result of the breakdown of old red blood cells. Prehepatic bilirubin is associated with the destruction of red blood cells.	Have other tests been done for the liver?
Post hepatic, conjugated, glucosuria, and direct reacting are the same.	Post hepatic 0.1 – 1.2 mg/dl	Increased levels may be seen in the newborn with an immature liver, or when there is a breakdown of red blood cells that the liver cannot handle. Increased levels of post hepatic may be seen in hepatitis or cirrhosis of the liver.	
Calcium	9 – 11 mg/dl	May be decreased with diarrhea, infections and kidney failure. May be elevated with fractures, exercise and some tumors.	Low levels may cause twitching or spasms. Foods high in calcium are milk products and protein.

Lab Value	Normal Ranges	Significance	What to ask? And Consider
Cardiac Troponin-I	Below 0.6 ng/ml	Provides a means for determining long-term risk after a heart attack. It is a very sensitive index for damage to the heart muscle.	Did a heart attack occur? What is the expected outcome if one did occur?
CEA Antigen	Nonsmokers below 2.5 ng/ml. Smokers below 5 ng/ml	This test is done to monitor the treatment for colon or pancreatic cancers. Elevated levels are seen with a number of different cancers.	An elevated level doesn't necessarily indicate the person has cancer.
Cerebro spinal fluid (CSF)	Clear and without bacteria.	The test is done via a procedure called a spinal tap or lumbar puncture to look for bacteria, bleeding, or abnormal cells in the spinal fluid.	The patient may need to lie flat for 4-8 hours after the procedure and may have a headache.
Cholesterol **LDL** **HDL**	Below 200 LDL – 60-160 mg/dl HDL 29-77 mg/dl	May be elevated with cardiac disease, liver problems, low thyroid, and diabetes. HDL is considered a friendly lipid. Problems occur with High LDL and low HDL.	Avoid foods with saturated fats and sugar.

Lab Value	Normal Ranges	Significance	What to ask? And Consider
Cold Agglutinins	1:8 antibody titer	May be elevated in certain pneumonias, flu, or liver problems.	Most persons have an antibody titer level, but older adults and those with viral infections may have a higher level.
CPK or CK creatine phosphokinaseor creatine kinase (CK)	20 – 135 IU	Mostly done to look for damage to the heart as is seen in a heart attack. When there is a heart attack (M.I.), the heart muscle releases CPK into the blood within the first 48 hours. Values return to normal in about 3 days.	Levels can also be elevated with injections and vigorous exercise.
Drug Levels - Acetamino-phen (Tylenol)	5 - 20 mcg/ml is therapeutic	Liver toxicity is likely with levels above 200 mg/L 4 hours post-ingestion	Tylenol should be taken as directed. Overdose can cause liver failure.
Drug Levels - Phenobarbital	15-40 mg/L	To verify that patient is getting enough medication.	Ask if dosages need to be altered.
Drug Level – Digoxin (Lanoxin)	0.5 – 2 ng/ml therapeutic	This test is ordered to monitor drug levels to see if the patient is getting enough medication.	When the level is toxic, heart rate may be low; there may be nausea or visual disturbances.

155

Lab Value	Normal Ranges	Significance	What to ask? And Consider
Drug Level – Phenytoin (Dilantin)	10 - 20 ug/ml therapeutic	To monitor phenytoin (Dilantin) levels.	Toxic levels may manifest as symptoms of slurred speech, jerking of the eyes, tiredness, rash, or confusion.
Drug Level – Gentamicin	<2 mcg/ml predose, 4-8 mcg/ml 1 hour post dose	Toxicity may result in hearing loss or kidney failure.	If you see changes, ask if lab tests have been done.
Drug Level – Lithium	0.8-1.2 mEq/L therapeutic	To identify Lithium toxicity.	Patients on lithium need adequate fluid and salt intake.
Drug Level – Theophylline Aminophylline	5 - 20 mg/L	To monitor theophylline levels.	Levels that are too high may increase heart rate.
ESR or sed rate	0 – 20 mm/hour	Erythrocyte sedimentation rate. May indicate inflam-matory process, tissue damage or infection.	If this test is elevated, ask if other tests should be done.
FDP Fibrin degradation products	2 – 10 mcg/ml	This test aids in the diagnosis of disseminated intravascular coagulation (DIC), a very serious situation that causes simultaneous clotting and bleeding in areas of the body.	This is a very serious diagnosis and usually requires intensive care nursing.

Lab Value	Normal Ranges	Significance	What to ask? And Consider
GGT gamma-glutamyl transpeptidase	4 – 23 IU	This is an enzyme found in the liver and used for detecting liver problems. The GGT levels will increase after 12 – 24 hours of heavy alcoholic drinking and may remain increased for 2 to 3 weeks after alcohol intake stops.	The test may be done for someone who is entering an alcohol rehabilitation program.
GTT, OGTT – Glucose Tolerance	Fasting 70-110 ½ hour below 160 1 hour below 170 2 hours below 125 3 hours 70-110	This test is used to confirm the diagnosis for diabetes mellitus. A solution (tastes like coke syrup) is swallowed or given via I.V.; blood sugar levels are checked at regular intervals to see how the body metabolizes the solution.	If diabetes is a new diagnosis, ask to speak to an educator to learn as much as possible about the disease.

Lab Value	Normal Ranges	Significance	What to ask? And Consider
Hemoglobin A1c (Hgb A1C or Hb A1C)	Nondiabetic 2-5% Diabetic control 2.5-6%	Also called glycosylated hemoglobin. This is one of the best tests to monitor the effectiveness of diabetic therapy and patient compliance. It is representative of the average blood glucose level over a 1 to 4 month time.	Reinforce for family members the importance of complying with insulin, diet, and glucose monitoring.
Lipase	20-180 IU/l	To test for acute pancreatitis.	Is there a problem with the pancreas? Have other tests been done?
Occult Blood (tested in stool)	Negative	This test is done to detect blood in the stool or feces. A smear of stool is taken and tested for blood. Stools that look like tar may have blood.	Iron preparations can cause dark-looking stool.
Platelet Count	150,000 – 400,000 mm3	Platelets are basic elements in the blood that promote clotting. Low counts place the patient at risk for bleeding.	If low, bleeding may be a concern. Be gentle with tooth brushing.

Lab Value	Normal Ranges	Significance	What to ask? And Consider
PSA – Prostate-specific antigen	0-4 ng/ml	Aids in the diagnosis of prostate cancer for men who have benign prostate enlargement.	Rectal exams are also done to feel for an enlarged prostate gland.
RBC count	4.2 – 6.2 million/mm3	The RBC contains hemoglobin, which carries oxygen. The RBC count is a reflection of oxygen-carrying capacity.	The components of the RBC are also checked to help classify anemias.
Reticulocyte Count	0.5 – 1.5%	This is an indicator of bone marrow activity and is used for diagnosing anemias.	Can we bring in food from home? What foods might help?
Thyroid Studies	TSH (0.35 – 5.5 mcg/IU/ml) T4 (4.5-11.5 mcg/dl) T3 (80-200 ng/dl)	TSH – thyroid stimulating hormone T4 – thyroxine T3 – tri-iodothyronine; A normal or elevated TSH level and a decreased T4 level could be due to thyroid dysfunction.	Signs of high thyroid are nervousness, fast heart rate, and weight loss. Signs of low thyroid are fatigue, dry skin, and thin hair.
Triglycerides	10 – 160 mg/dl depending on age	To monitor triglyceride levels. Triglycerides are a major contributor to arterial disease.	With high levels, avoid eating excess sugars or carbohydrates.

Appendix G: Chapter 6
Additional Diagnostic Tests

Test Name	Description and Use	Where Done	Comments
Arthroscopy	To examine the inside of a joint.	Usually in surgery.	A small incision is made for the scope.
Barium Enema	To detect disorders of the large intestine. The bowel is usually cleared first with enemas or laxatives.	Radiology.	An enema tube is placed in the rectum. A dye (barium) is given via enema so that the x-ray can take a picture.
Bone Density	To evaluate the bone mineral density and identify early and progressive osteoporosis.	Radiology	This is a very useful screening tool.
Bronchoscopy	To inspect the upper airway or remove foreign bodies.	Surgery or special lab.	A large scope is inserted through the nose or mouth to view the lungs. Medications will be given to help decrease anxiety. Usually performed under local anesthetic.

Test Name	Description and Use	Where Done	Comments
Cardiac Catheterization	A type of Angiography to view the arteries that supply the heart, look at heart size, structure, valves and pressures.	Catheterization lab, radiology.	A long catheter is threaded from the groin into the heart. The right side of the heart is viewed from a vein, the left side from an artery. You will need to lie flat in bed for some time.
Cholangiography	Looks at the liver, bile ducts and gallbladder.	Radiology	Patient will usually be in bed for 6 hours after the procedure.
Gallbladder Series	To look for stones or tumor, or obstruction in the gallbladder.	Radiology	There are times when the test needs to be repeated.
Cystoscopy	This test provides a direct visualization of the bladder and the tube that takes urine out of the body (urethra). The test looks for stones and tumors in the bladder.	Surgery, special labs	The procedure is done under local or general anesthetic. There may be some pressure, burning, or discomfort during the test.
Echocardiogram	Done to identify heart size, structure, and function. The test also evaluates coronary artery disease and function of the heart chambers.	Bedside, office, or cardiology department.	May be done with contrast (dye injected) or after exercise on a treadmill or bicycle.

Test Name	Description and Use	Where Done	Comments
EEG, electroence-phalography	Done to detect seizure disorders, brain tumor, abscess or bleeding in the head. Also done to help determine brain death. Electrodes are attached to the head.	Bedside, office or in a specialized department.	Hair should be clean without oil or hair spray. Does not cause any type of electrical shock.
Fluoroscopy	The purpose of this test is to view the functions of organs in motion.	Radiology	Causes no discomfort.
Gastric Analysis	The test examines stomach secretions. A tube is placed in the nose into the stomach to withdraw fluid. There are procedures where this can be done without a tube, but the results don't reveal as much.	Radiology	Patient will be asked to swallow the tube. The procedure can be uncomfortable.
Holter Monitoring	To identify heart rhythm problems. A cardiac monitor with electrodes is placed on the chest. The patient carries a tape type device that records events that occur with the heart.	Monitor attached in an office or cardiology department.	The patient will need to keep a diary of events and push an event marker during the day, such as palpitations or chest pain. Data is analyzed at a later date with the tape data.

Test Name	Description and Use	Where Done	Comments
Laparoscopy	To visualize the abdominal and pelvic organs. A small incision is made in the abdomen. A scope is inserted to view the area.	Surgery	Patient may complain of gas pains after the procedure.
Mammography	Used to screen for breast masses and look for tumors or cysts.	Radiology	May cause discomfort, as the breast is compressed during the exam.
Myelogram	This is an exam of the spinal cord using air or a contrast to view. Used to detect spinal regions.	Radiology	Patient usually remains flat for 6 to 8 hours. Usually nothing to eat 4 to 6 hours before the test.
Nuclear Scans	Done on various body parts utilizing safe radioactive materials or isotopes.	Radiology, Nuclear Medicine	Radiation amounts are usually less than a standard x-ray. Test takes 30 minutes to 1 hour and may need to be repeated.
PET (positron emission tomography)	A noninvasive test to measure the heart, brain, lungs or internal organs.	Radiology, Nuclear Medicine	Nothing by mouth for 4 to 6 hours. Velcro straps may be used to hold body parts still.
Proctosigmoidoscopy **proctoscopy** **sigmoidoscopy**	An examination of the anus, rectum and sigmoid colon. A long tube is inserted into the rectum.	GI Lab or Radiology	There may be some discomfort, but should not cause severe pain. Take slow, deep breaths during the procedure to help relax.

Test Name	Description and Use	Where Done	Comments
Pulmonary Function Tests	Used to check for various lung diseases. Often done for a baseline. Also done to assess lung and respiratory function.	Cardio-pulmonary Department or in the office	Patient will be asked to take deep breaths and perform forced exhalations to measure values.
Radioactive iodine (RAI) uptake test	Used to determine metabolic activity of the thyroid gland. Helps to diagnose increased or decreased thyroid activity.	Radiology, Nuclear Medicine	The patient may be asked to return to nuclear medicine at very specific times. The radioactive substance is very low dosage and doesn't harm others.
Retrograde Pyelography, Retrograde pyelogram	Views the urinary tract. A dye is injected into the tubes that flow from the kidneys to the bladder. May look for kidney problems or stones.	Radiology	An iodine-based dye is used. Be sure to tell the technician and doctor if you are allergic to seafood or iodine.
Skin Testing	Used to determine present or past exposure to an infectious organism. One of the most common tests is for tuberculosis. A small amount of substance is injected into the inner arm.	Test may be performed in the office or anywhere in the hospital.	The test must be read during the stated time. A positive does not always indicate active infection. It does indicate the organism is present, but may be active or dormant.

Test Name	Description and Use	Where Done	Comments
Sleep Studies (polysom-nography) PSG	Used to determine the cause of sleep disorders, most often sleep apnea. Electrodes will be attached to the head, chest and legs in a controlled environment.	Usually at a sleep center. Some agencies perform the test in the home.	Heart monitoring, brain monitoring, and oxygen saturation (small device on the finger) may be done at the same time.
Stress/ exercise, treadmill testing	Done to screen for coronary artery disease and for developing a cardiac rehabilitation program. The test may also be done to determine the effect of drug dosing. Some stress tests use drugs to increase heart rate rather than exercise.	Cardio-pulmonary department	Patient may need to exercise on a treadmill or bicycle to increase the heart rate. Comfortable clothes and tennis shoes with socks must be worn.
Thoracoscopy	Used to obtain biopsy specimens or remove fluid from the chest area. A tube is inserted into the chest area to look at the lungs and chest area.	Surgery	Patient will have anesthesia and a chest tube with a drainage system will be placed after the test. Patient will need to be monitored in the hospital.

Test Name	Description and Use	Where Done	Comments
Ultrasound, Sonogram	Visualizes various body structures. The test, which is non-invasive, may evaluate blood flow in arteries and veins, look for cysts, tumors or stones.	Radiology, at bedside	An oil or lubricant is applied to the skin and the probe is moved with light pressure back and forwards.
Venogram	An x-ray exam of the deep leg veins after a dye is injected to look for clots.	Radiology	There might be a burning sensation after the dye is injected. Tell the physician and technician if there are allergies to seafood or iodine.
Ventilation Scan	This is a nuclear scan of the lungs. The patient inhales a mixture of gases. Evaluates problems related to blood flow to the lungs such as a blood clot.	Radiology	The amount of radioactive gas is minimal.

Appendix H: Chapter 9
Discharge Questionnaires

48 hours before discharge

Task	Completed?	Questions?
Has discharge been discussed with the family members who need to know?		
Have written and verbal advice been given to the patient?		
Have arrangements been confirmed?		
Does the caregiver understand how to use special equipment?		
Have transfer arrangements been made?		
Has there been training on the hospital equipment?		
Have friends or family brought clothes to go home in?		

Day of Discharge

Task	Completed	Questions
Has access to the home been arranged?		
Have medication instructions been given to the patient and the caregiver?		
Have prescriptions been obtained?		
Did someone pick up the prescriptions?		
Did the nursing staff provide medications before going home?		
Have community agencies been contacted?		
Is the necessary equipment in place in the home?		
Has a follow-up physician appointment been made?		
Is transportation confirmed?		
Has the patient been given a list of when to call the physician?		
Has the patient or caregivers been given a list of what situations would constitute a 911 call?		
Have financial obligations been met?		

References

Topic	Description	Resource or Web Site
Discharge	Checklist	http://www.publications.doh.gov.uk/hospitaldischarge/ch5app2.htm
Discharge	Choosing Ambulatory Care	http://www.jcaho.org/general+public/making+better+choices/helping+you+choose/ac.htm
Discharge	Choosing Assisted Living	http://www.jcaho.org/general+public/making+better+choices/helping+you+choose/assisted+living.htm
Discharge	Choosing Behavioral Health Care	http://www.jcaho.org/general+public/making+better+choices/helping+you+choose/bhc.htm
Discharge	Helping You Choose Quality Behavioral Health-care	http://www.jcaho.org/general+public/making+better+choices/helping+you+choose/bhc.htm
Discharge	Helping You Choose Quality Homecare and Hospice	http://www.jcaho.org/general+public/making+better+choices/helping+you+choose/hc.htm
Discharge	Options	http://www.ottawahospital.on.ca/hp/dept/socialwork/discharge-e.asp#options
Drugs	FDA site	http://vm.cfsan.fda.gov
Hospice	National Hospice and Palliative Care Organization	http://www.nhpco.org/i4a/pages/index.cfm?pageid=3254&openpage=3254
Hospital	Choosing Hospital Care	http://www.jcaho.org/general+public/making+better+choices/helping+you+choose/hos.htm
Hospital	Helping You Choose Quality Ambulatory Care	http://www.jcaho.org/general+public/making+better+choices/helping+you+choose/ac.htm

Topic	Description	Resource or Web Site
Hospital	Patient Questions in Critical Care	http://www.acs.ohio-state.edu/units/ osuhosp/patedu/Materials/PDFDocs/ general/choices-for.pdf
Hospital	Safety	Consumer Reports, January 2003, How Safe is Your Hospital? What You Need to Know that Hospitals Don't Reveal.
Hospitals	Consumer Reports Article	http://www.consumerreports.org/main/ detailv2.jsp?CONTENT%3C%3Ecnt_i d=297913&FOLDER%3C%3Efolder_ id=162687
Lab Values	Lab Values	Fischbach, Frances, A Manual of Laboratory & Diagnostic Tests, 6th Edition, 2000, Lippincott
Legal	Advanced Directives	http://www.partnershipforcaring.org/ Advance/faq_set.html
Legal	Choosing Long-Term Care	http://www.jcaho.org/general+public/ making+better+choices/ helping+you+choose/ltc.htm
Legal	Durable Power of Attorney for Healthcare	http://www.ilrg.com/forms/states/ca-powerofattorneyhealth.html
Legal Forms	Advance Directives	http://www.partnershipforcaring.org/ Advance/index.html
Legal Forms	Advance Directives	http://www.partnershipforcaring.org/ Advance/faq_set.html
Legal Forms	Living Will	http://www.ilrg.com/forms/livingwill. html
Legal Forms	Living Will Example for California	http://www.ilrg.com/forms/states/ca-livingwill.html
Medical Terminology	Abbreviations	(http://courses.smsu.edu/jas188f/690/ medslpterm.html)

Topic	Description	Resource or Web Site
Medical Terminology	Terms	Masters, Regina & Glylys, Barbara. Medical Terminology: A Medical Specialties Approach with Patient Records. F.A. Davis, Philadelphia, 2003.
Nursing Skills	Basic Skills	Roe, Susan, Delmar's Clinical Nursing Skills & Concepts, Thompson, Delmar Learning, 2003
Nursing Skills	Basic Skills	White, Lois and Duncan, Gena. Medical-Surgical Nursing, An Integrated Approach. Second Edition. Thompson, Delmar Learning, 2002.
Nutrition	Nutrition in wound healing	http://www.abbott.ca/eng/health/woundcare.pdf
Nutrition	FDA	http://www.cfsan.fda.gov/~dms/fdsp-diet.html
Nutrition	Food and Drug Home Instructions	West Hills Hospital and Medical Center, Patient Handout
Nutrition	Foods High in Protein	http://www.geocities.com/Heartland/Plains/9847/protein.html
Nutrition	Nutrition in hospitalized patients (animals)	http://www.vspn.org/Library/Rounds/VSPN_VSPN011116.htm
Nutrition	Nutritional assessment of Hospitalized Patients: Overlooked Area of Lab testing	http://www.aacc.org/cln/features/98features/feb98feat.html
Nutrition	Poor Hospital Nutrition is killing elderly patients	http://www.wcanews.com/archives/1999/aug/aug99d.htm
Nutrition	Poor Nutrition in Hospitalized Seniors	http://www.healthandage.com/Home/gm=6!gid2=884
Nutrition	Protein Malnutrition	http://www.healthatoz.com/healthatoz/Atoz/ency/protein-energy_malnutrition.html

Topic	Description	Resource or Web Site
Nutrition	Special Diets	Manual of Clinical Dietetics, 6th Edition, American Dietetic Association, 2000.
Nutrition	Weight-Gaining Recipes	www.caretody.com
Psychological Resources	Grief	http://www.mydogandi.com/living\death\death1.htm
Psychological Resources	Maslow's Hierarchy	Gorman, Raines and Sultan, Psycho-social Nursing for General Patient Care, second edition, 2002, F.A. Davis, Philadelphia
Sentinel Events	JCAHO sentinel events 2003	http://www.jcaho.org/accredited+organizations/office+based+surgery/sentinel+events/se_stats.pdf
Speak Up	"Speak Up" suggestions	http://www.nursingworld.org
Speak Up	JCAHO Accreditation	http://www.nursingworld.org/press-rel/2002/pr0318.htm
Speak Up	JCAHO Accreditation	http://www.jcaho.org/general+public/patient+safety/speak+up/speak+up.htm
Speak Up	JCAHO Preventing Errors in Your Care	http://www.jcaho.org

Notes

Notes

Notes